AF835571

Toxic oil syndrome

Mass food poisoning in Spain

World Health Organization
Regional Office for Europe
Copenhagen

Toxic oil syndrome

Mass food poisoning in Spain

Report on a WHO meeting
Madrid, 21–25 March 1983

ISBN 92 890 1021 5

© World Health Organization 1984

Publications of the World Health Organization enjoy copyright protection in accordance with the provisions of Protocol 2 of the Universal Copyright Convention. For rights of reproduction or translation, in part or *in toto,* of publications issued by the WHO Regional Office for Europe application should be made to the Regional Office for Europe, Scherfigsvej 8, DK-2100 Copenhagen Ø, Denmark. The Regional Office welcomes such applications.

The designations employed and the presentation of the material in this publication do not imply the expression of any opinion whatsoever on the part of the Secretariat of the World Health Organization concerning the legal status of any country, territory, city or area or of its authorities, or concerning the delimitation of its frontiers or boundaries.

The mention of specific companies or of certain manufacturers' products does not imply that they are endorsed or recommended by the World Health Organization in preference to others of a similar nature that are not mentioned. Errors and omissions excepted, the names of proprietary products are distinguished by initial capital letters.

The views expressed in this publication are those of the participants in the meeting and do not necessarily represent the decisions or the stated policy of the World Health Organization.

Printed in England.

CONTENTS

EDITORS

Philippe Grandjean
Department of Environmental Medicine
Odense University
Denmark

Stanislaw Tarkowski
WHO Regional Office for Europe
Copenhagen, Denmark

CONTRIBUTORS

V. Faro
Ramón y Cajal Centre
Madrid, Spain

J.G. Rigau-Perez
Centers for Disease Control
Atlanta, GA, USA

G.K. Koch
Unilever Research Laboratorium
Vlaardingen, Netherlands

M. Serrano-Rios
Ramón y Cajal Centre
Madrid, Spain

J.M. Tabuenca Oliver
Clinical Commission
National Programme for the Toxic Syndrome
Madrid, Spain

Foreword

On 1 May 1981, the first case of a disease, later to be designated "toxic oil syndrome", was encountered in Spain. Physicians were immediately struck by the disease's unique clinical appearance which separated it from any other known disease condition. Evidence quickly accumulated to indicate that the disease was environmentally induced, but the critical cornerstone on which to base prevention and treatment was still missing: which environmental factor was the cause? Answering this important question rapidly became an acute necessity, as thousands of patients began to overcrowd the hospitals in Madrid and the north-western parts of Spain. Several pieces of evidence pointed towards the ingestion of adulterated edible oil, containing refined denatured rapeseed oil, as being the causal factor. Emergency responses, in particular public warnings and the recall of suspect oil, were then initiated by the public health authorities.

Several characteristics of this tragic event relate to food safety and environmental health concerns worldwide. The toxic oil syndrome (TOS) was immediately recognized as a new disease; had this not been the case, many more people might have become ill before its cause was identified, or even suspected. Unlike with many environmentally induced diseases that mimic common syndromes and are not easily related to a specific, preventable cause, the diagnosis of TOS was straightforward. We can only speculate what would have happened if the environmental factor had been less obvious. Since the acute effects occurred within a week or so of exposure to the clandestine oil, problems related to latency period or induction time were of minor importance in the search for a causal factor. The long-term effects have yet to be defined in detail.

After the suspect oil had been traced to a specific food oil company, preventive and remedial action was rather clearcut. By contrast, most other environmental exposure occurs through various pathways, at irregular levels or intervals, and in conjunction with other factors that may interfere with the observed effects. Thus, the occurrence of TOS in Spain, though catastrophic, followed a relatively simple chain of events.

The lessons to be learned from this type of avoidable tragedy therefore have serious and far-reaching significance for preventive action in environmental health in general. First, the immediate need for stricter and more effective food safety enforcement is imperative. Second, an improved epidemiological programme and a strengthening of toxicological resources are necessary. The training of physicians and other health professionals in these areas must be intensified, and a multidisciplinary approach to preventive environmental medicine needs to be further developed. Finally, plans for emergency response should be reviewed and improved. It should be stressed that although these recommendations relate to a particular incident in one country, they are of great importance and relevance to all countries, owing to the ubiquity of environmental hazards.

The early recognition by the Government of Spain that the importance of TOS extended beyond national borders to general considerations of human health led to prompt international involvement and encouraged the scientific community in its efforts to pinpoint the cause of the disease and initiate preventive and rehabilitative measures. At the request of the Spanish authorities, WHO has been involved in TOS since the early phase of the disease. Through WHO, the knowledge and experience of clinicians, epidemiologists and toxicologists have been brought to bear on this important health problem. In addition to the efforts made within Spain, scientific research contributions have been made by groups in other countries, namely: Unilever Research Laboratorium, Vlaardingen, Netherlands; Medical Research Council Laboratories, Toxicology Unit, Carshalton, United Kingdom; Centers for Disease Control, Atlanta, Georgia, United States; and National Institute of Environmental Health Sciences/National Toxicology Program, Research Triangle Park, North Carolina, United States. These contributions and the efforts of those who contributed their expertise to the WHO Working Group on the Toxic Oil Syndrome, held in Madrid on 21–25 March 1983, are hereby acknowledged. This publication presents the report of the Working Group, as well as additional scientific reviews of specific aspects of TOS.

Many questions concerning TOS are still unanswered. In particular, the specific substance or substances in the oil that caused the disease have not yet been identified. This aspect also deserves international attention and may only be resolved through cooperation among research institutions in several countries.

J.I. Waddington

Director, Environmental Health Service
WHO Regional Office for Europe

Introduction

In early May 1981 a previously unknown disease syndrome broke out in Spain, primarily in Madrid and in the provinces north-west of Madrid. The epidemic reached a peak by mid-June, when over 600 daily hospital admissions due to the disease were recorded. Once illegally sold denatured rapeseed oil had been identified as the most probable cause, an exchange of the suspect cooking oil with pure olive oil was initiated by the Government. The epidemic then faded away, although chronic cases continued to be discovered. Many cases of the disease were severe and needed intensive care. By March 1983 a total of 340 deaths had occurred, the total number of cases recorded exceeded 20 000, and a small number of patients were still in intensive care. The severity of this epidemic and its associated important medical and toxicological aspects prompted an international collaborative effort to establish precise diagnostic criteria, the mechanisms of pathogenesis, epidemiological characteristics and the identity of the causal agent or agents. In addition, the implications for the prevention of similar incidents needed to be assessed.

The WHO Working Group on the Toxic Oil Syndrome was held at the Ministry of Health and Consumer Affairs in Madrid, from 21 to 25 March 1983. The meeting was opened by Mrs C. Salanueva, Director-General of the National Programme for the Toxic Syndrome, who stressed that the results of the meeting would be of considerable importance to the continued work of the National Programme. Mr J.I. Waddington welcomed the participants on behalf of the WHO Regional Director for Europe, and reviewed the involvement of WHO at the request of the Government of Spain. Several consultation meetings had been arranged, and WHO consultants had visited Spain and made recommendations about continued efforts. The Working Group was planned in close cooperation with the Spanish authorities. On the basis of toxicological, clinical and epidemiological data, it was hoped that specific conclusions would be reached by the participants. In addition, the meeting should note the general lessons learned so that similar tragedies in Spain and other countries could be prevented. Dr S. Tarkowski presented the scope and purpose of the meeting, noting that numerous documents had already been distributed and that a critical assessment of the background information and the current situation would be pertinent. Gaps in knowledge and priority problems should be identified. Conclusions and recommendations should focus on both practical and theoretical questions and on the wider aspects of future preventive action. The meeting comprised a plenary session to review current information, and three subgroups on epidemiology, clinical observations and pathology, and toxicology.

Mrs C. Salanueva was elected Chairman, Professor R. Goulding and Dr A. Portera Sánchez were elected Vice-Chairmen, and Professor P. Grandjean was elected Rapporteur.

1

Review of investigations and findings

Epidemiology and Etiology

Owing to its relationship to the ingestion of contaminated cooking oil (see Annex 1), the disease was named the toxic oil syndrome (TOS) by the Working Group. Without doubt, this disease is a new entity. The major epidemiological aspects of TOS may be described under five headings: time of occurrence, geographic occurrence, demographic characteristics, association with oil use, and possible causal agents in the oil.

Time of occurrence

The epidemic was explosive and abrupt. The new disease was first encountered on 1 May 1981 in an 8-year-old boy dying from acute pulmonary insufficiency. He belonged to a Madrid family of eight, six of whom eventually fell ill. The epidemic reached a peak by mid-June when 600 daily hospital admissions due to TOS were recorded. During May and June about 10 000 cases were seen in hospitals (Fig. 1), and 80 deaths occurred in the acute phase of the disease (Fig. 2). Clinical impression suggests that the severity of the disease may have been greater earlier in the epidemic than it was later. Over the next six months only 2600 new cases were discovered, with most reportedly in a chronic phase, and a similar number of TOS patients were readmitted. Coinciding with the sharp decrease in the incidence of acute cases of the disease from late June was the announcement by the Minister of Health and Consumer Affairs on 26 June that pure olive oil would be substituted for suspect toxic oil beginning on 30 June at the latest. Although a causal relationship is not proven by this apparent association, the withdrawal of the oil offers a possible explanation of the sudden disappearance of acute cases, and no other possibility has been substantiated by supporting evidence.

Geographic occurrence

Cases of TOS appeared first in Madrid and then spread to the provinces largely north-west of the capital (Fig. 3). The epidemic was mainly confined to the 14 provinces indicated in Fig. 4 and 5; fewer than 200 cases were seen in other parts of the country, and most of these originated elsewhere. No

Fig. 1. New cases and readmissions of TOS by week

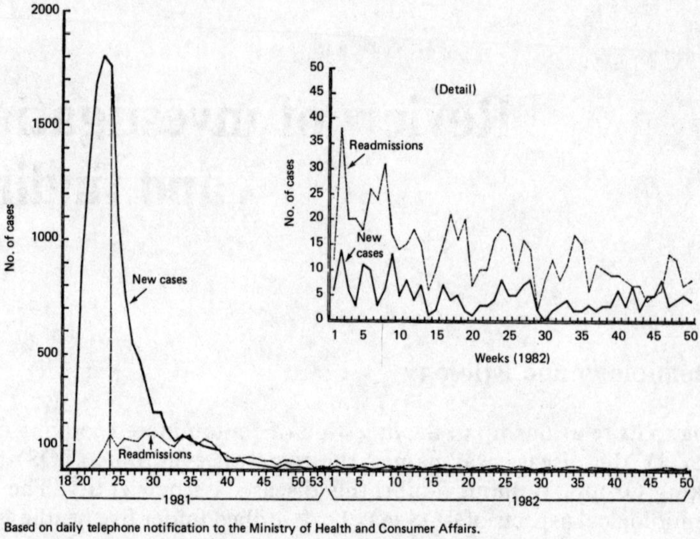

Based on daily telephone notification to the Ministry of Health and Consumer Affairs.

Source: Boletín epidemiológico semanal, **1561**: 273–275 (1983).

Fig. 2. TOS deaths by week

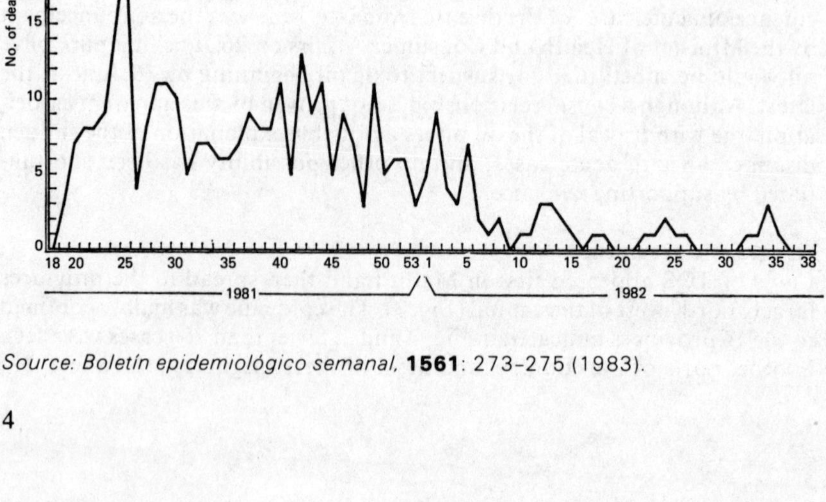

Source: Boletín epidemiológico semanal, **1561**: 273–275 (1983).

Fig. 3. Date of first recorded cases of TOS in 14 provinces

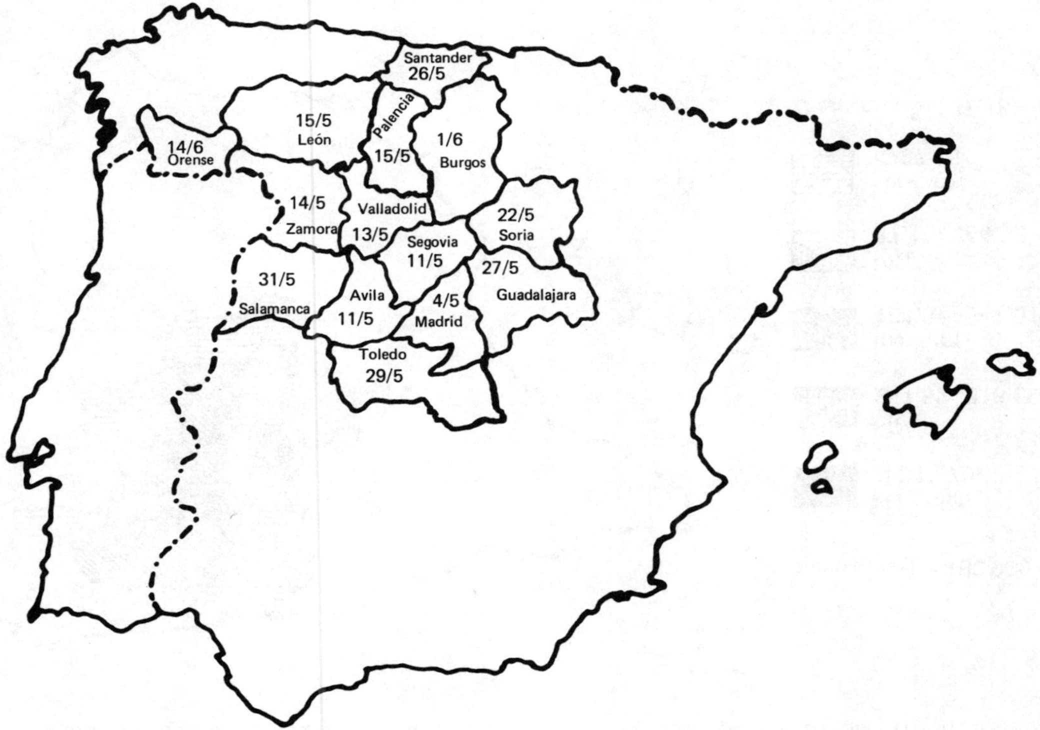

Source: *Boletín epidemiológico semanal,* **1482**: 129–131 (1981).

Fig. 4. Total incidence of TOS per 100 000 inhabitants in 14 provinces with more than 12 recorded cases, as of October 1982, when 18 893 cases were recorded in these provinces

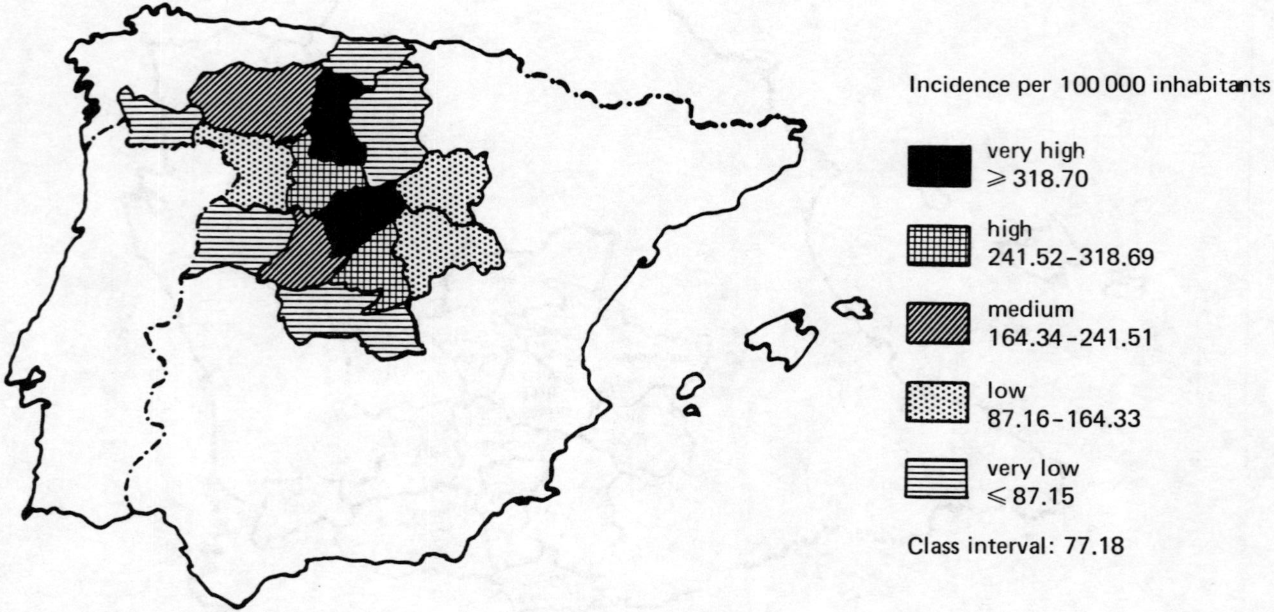

Source: Boletín epidemiológico semanal, **1565**: 301–303 (1983).

Fig. 5. Mortality from TOS per 100 000 inhabitants in the 14 provinces indicated in Fig. 4, based on 336 deaths

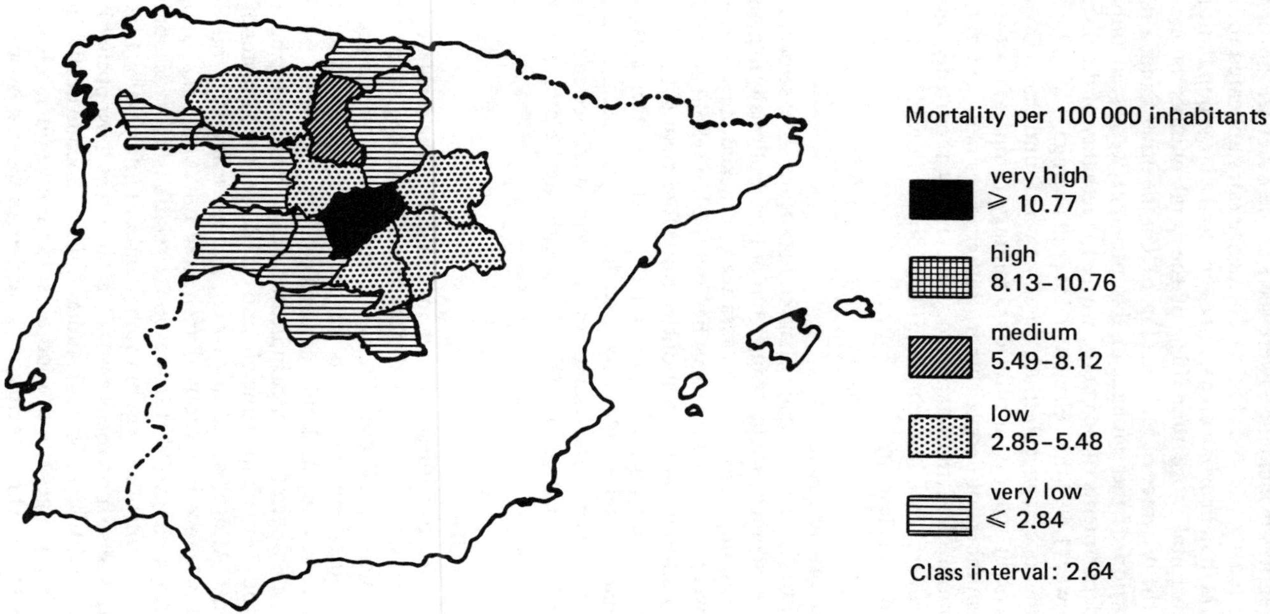

Source: Boletín epidemiológico semanal, **1565**: 301–303 (1983).

case was found to originate outside Spain. The incidence rates, as calculated 18 months after the outbreak, were about 300 cases per 100 000 inhabitants in the provinces of Segovia, Palencia, Valladolid and Madrid, while somewhat or much lower incidences were seen in the other ten north-western provinces primarily affected (Fig. 4). Incidence rates appeared to be much higher in rural than in urban areas, but owing to the large population in and around the capital more than 70% of the total number of cases were recorded in the province of Madrid (Fig. 6). On the other hand, a relatively large proportion of the patients in this province were seen only in the outpatient departments of hospitals, where the lethality of the disease was somewhat lower (1.6%) than elsewhere (overall average, 1.8%). Looking at the geographic occurrence in more detail, it was found that TOS was not more frequent in schools, institutions, military camps and other places where large numbers of people gather. Rather, cases belonged to the same household more often than expected. One survey reportedly linked the location of several case households to the route followed by a particular itinerant food oil salesman.

Demographic characteristics

With regard to the demographic characteristics, the disease occurred primarily in lower socioeconomic groups, but only exceptionally in gypsies and the poorest. Family members of cases were attacked surprisingly often, while there were no secondary cases beyond the household circle. No case occurred in children under six months old. More than 60% of the cases recorded were female (Fig. 7). In addition, the mortality in females was twice as high as that in males, reflecting a slightly higher lethality in females (Fig. 8). In both men and women, the highest incidence rates occurred between 31 and 60 years of age (Fig. 7), but the age relationship was not striking.

Association with oil use

Several etiological hypotheses were launched during the early weeks of the epidemic. Later, some positive evidence from microbiological studies led to the announcement on 21 May that mycoplasma infection was the cause of the disease. Questionnaire studies suggested the possibility of a food-mediated intoxication, and this conclusion was broadcast on 1 June. Further epidemiological evidence indicated a close relationship between the disease and the use of clandestine oil, and on 10 June the Minister of Health and Consumer Affairs issued a warning against using such oil. Raw oil appeared to be more hazardous than heated oil. Additional supporting evidence, with a suggested dose–response relationship, was obtained in successive case-control studies, but some degree of information bias cannot be excluded because food oil as a possible cause was most probably public knowledge after 10 June. Several studies pointed unequivocally, however, to the cause being ingestion of food oil sold as olive oil at a low price by itinerant salesmen. This conclusion is further supported by a number of somewhat anecdotal case reports or studies of clusters. Although other

Fig. 6. Number of TOS cases by province, as of October 1982

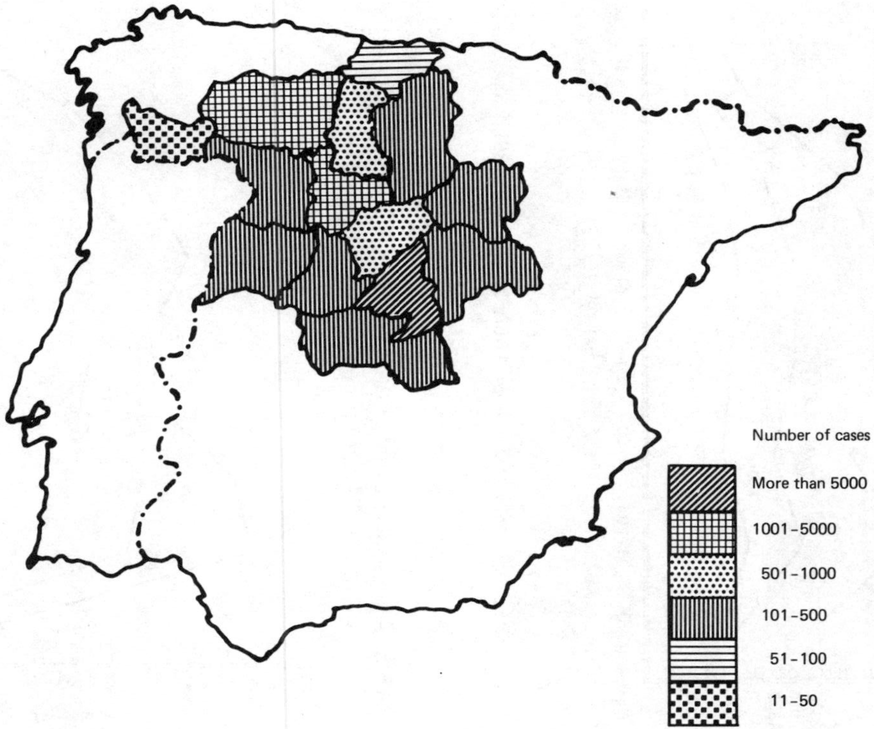

Source: *Boletín epidemiológico semanal,* **1565**: 301–303 (1983).

Fig. 7. Age and sex distribution of TOS patients recorded in the 14 provinces indicated in Fig. 4, as of September 1982

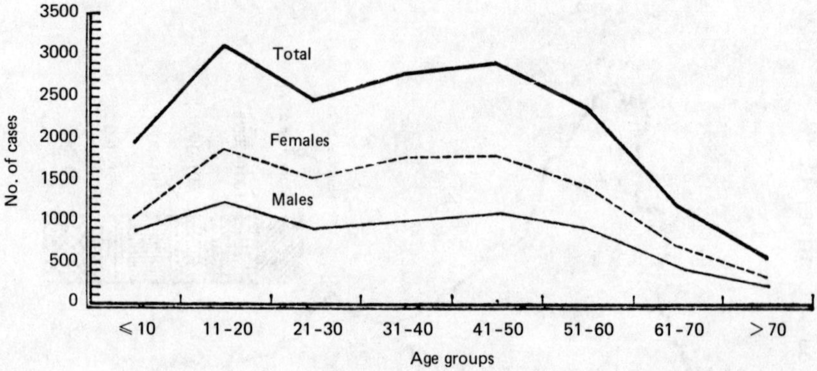

Source: Boletín epidemiológico semanal, **1562**: 281–283 (1983).

Fig. 8. Age and sex distribution of 336 TOS-related deaths in the 14 provinces indicated in Fig. 4

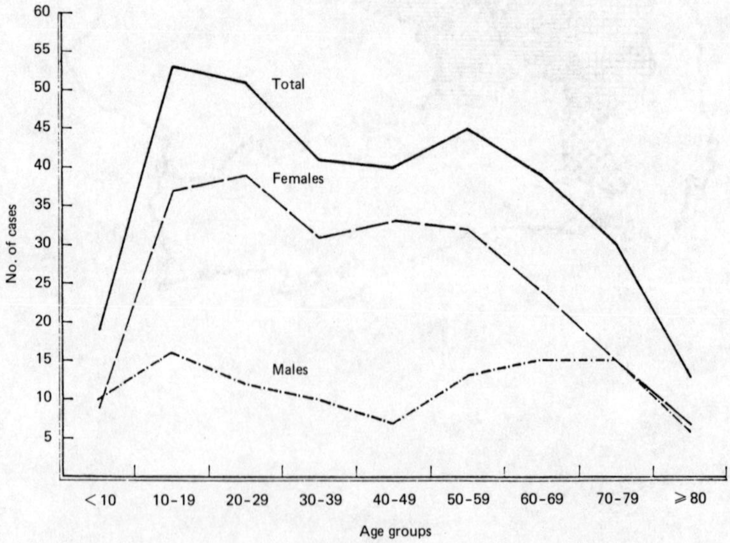

Source: Boletín epidemiológico semanal, **1564**: 293–295 (1983).

possibilities have been suggested, contaminated food oil appears to be the only likely cause.

Possible causal agents in the oil

The search for toxic agents in the oil has been largely futile. Investigations showed that rapeseed oil was imported and denatured, as required by law, with 2% aniline for industrial use. This oil was then de-denatured by a refining process that apparently removed almost all the aniline, and the oil was then mixed with 10–30% of other seed oils, about 30% of animal fats and up to 5% of a poor quality olive oil or, alternatively, chlorophyll to obtain the colour desired. The product was sold primarily in unlabelled 5-litre plastic containers through street vendors and itinerant salesmen. Early studies showed that there was no mineral oil or orthocresolphosphate in the product. In addition, erucic acid concentrations were very low, and maleic anhydride was not found in oil samples analysed. Other possibilities were explored without success. Three cases from Seville were traced to undiluted de-denatured rapeseed oil obtained directly from the refining facility. Although clandestine oil containing aniline may have been marketed in the past without catastrophic consequences, these cases strongly suggest that the cause of TOS was one or more components of this particular de-denatured rapeseed oil. Unfortunately, the unsolved problem is still the exact identity of these components.

Clinical Appearance

TOS consisted of a wide and unique variety of clinical symptoms, and virtually any tissue or organ appeared to be affected during some stage of the disease. The clinical picture varied considerably with time, and a division into acute and chronic phases seems justified.

The latency period from the first ingestion of contaminated oil appeared to vary somewhat, perhaps related to the dose absorbed and the frequency of ingestion. Scattered observations indicated a latency time of at least one week in adults, but a somewhat shorter period was seen in some children. During the latency period a prodromal stage may have occurred, as observed in some patients with eosinophilia before the development of symptoms. This suggestion was supported by the finding of an increased prevalence of eosinophilia in healthy members of households with TOS cases.

Acute phase

In the acute phase the clinical picture most frequently included fever, respiratory insufficiency with dyspnoea and cough, and exanthema (often of a pruritic nature). Other symptoms often encountered were nausea and vomiting, headache, muscle pains and diarrhoea. Further examination usually revealed the presence of noncardiogenic pulmonary oedema (sometimes with pleural effusion), eosinophilia and increased serum levels of immunoglobulin E (IgE). Most patients improved spontaneously; after about a week the fever disappeared and the radiographic changes in the lungs cleared away. Respiratory distress was the immediate cause of death in most cases of TOS mortality during the acute phase, i.e. in almost a quarter of all deaths in these patients. About 20% of the patients failed, despite corticosteroid treatment, to recover completely from pulmonary disease. Many of these cases later progressed into pulmonary arterial hypertension and respiratory insufficiency related to the motor weakness of the ventilatory musculature.

The skin changes varied in appearance from macules or papules to toxic eczema-like patches. The cheeks were often flushed, and this change was occasionally the only skin abnormality found. In most cases the cutaneous changes cleared in about two weeks. As described below, however, some patients later developed other skin changes.

Immunological alterations seen in the acute phase comprised marked eosinophilia, increased IgE, increased frequency of antinuclear, antipulmonary or antilymphocyte antibodies, and reduced numbers of thymus-derived lymphocytes. One laboratory reported specific IgE antibodies against fatty acid anilides, but the significance of this finding is difficult to assess. The immunological changes may not bear a direct relationship to the pathogenesis of TOS; rather, they may reflect a failure in the regulation of the immune system, possibly related to a primary toxic response. Few of the abnormalities subsisted, and the immunological picture appeared to change as the disease developed.

Some patients entered a transitional phase with the following symptoms: pulmonary arterial hypertension and mesenteric thrombosis; myalgia, cramps and muscle weakness with limited electromyographic changes; thrombocytopenia, eosinophilia, liver enzyme abnormalities, and antilymphocyte antibodies. While fever disappeared within a few weeks in most patients, the prevalence of eosinophilia increased during the same period and decreased only slowly during the transitional period when myalgia became an increasingly common symptom. Weakness and weight loss were also common features.

Chronic phase

The chronic phase was characterized by progressive muscle wasting, diffuse and symmetrical peripheral neuropathy, scleroderma-like skin lesions and the sicca syndrome. Most patients exhibited myalgia, cramps, paraesthesia, areflexia, muscular atrophy, muscle weakness and sensory deficits, while central nervous system changes were much less frequent. With time, the myalgia improved slightly but cramps, paraesthesia and sensory deficits worsened. Myoclonus and tremor became important features of the disease picture, occurring in about a quarter of the patients with chronic TOS. The considerable variability in the clinical appearance of these patients was striking. Electromyographic examinations showed spontaneous activity with a reduced interference pattern, reduced compound muscle action potential, and reduced or absent nerve action potential. Later, myoclonic bursts developed. Nerve conduction velocities exhibited moderate slowing. Muscle biopsy studies indicated severe neurogenic muscular atrophy. Nerve biopsies showed perineural fibrosis, patchy or total axonal loss, only occasional myelin lesions, but many vascular inflammatory infiltrates. Serum levels of creatinine phosphokinase were normal, and no abnormalities were found on cerebrospinal fluid examination, electroencephalography or computer-aided tomography of the brain.

Thus, this unique disease mainly showed a sensorimotor polyneuropathy of variable appearance. The pathogenesis is unclear but may be related to fibrosis of the perineural connective tissue and enteritis of the small vessels, possibly with subsequent axonal damage. Some evidence of neuronal damage suggests that a "dying-back" effect on the axons could occur. Direct toxic damage to the muscular tissue is also indicated. During the chronic phase scleroderma-like skin changes also developed, with increased collagen formation and signs of the sicca syndrome: reduced saliva production, atrophy of the parotid ducts on sialography, and round-cell infiltration of salivary gland tissue. Oesophageal function was often abnormal, and liver enzyme alterations frequently persisted. On the other hand, the thrombocytopenia and eosinophilia tended to normalize during this stage. In patients with the most severe symptoms the disease progressed towards undernutrition, endocrinological dysfunction, osteoporosis and other abnormalities that could be secondary to the direct effects described above.

Autopsy Findings

Twenty consecutive autopsies (of eleven patients in the acute and transitional phases, nine in the chronic phase) were performed in one of the hospitals in Madrid, and detailed pathology studies and biopsy results were reviewed.

Acute phase

During the acute phase the main pathological changes were found in the lungs: intense pulmonary interstitial oedema with only scanty inflammatory mononuclear infiltrates. Ultrastructural studies showed hydropic degeneration of pneumonocytes types I and II with desquamation of type I cells. The cause of death in this stage was respiratory failure. Blood vessels of every type and size located in almost any organ were affected by a non-necrotizing vasculitis, mainly in the intima. In addition, interstitial inflammatory infiltrates and/or fibrosis were seen in most organs. When the pulmonary changes of the acute phase had cleared, thromboembolic complication became the cause of death in patients in the transitional phase of TOS.

Chronic phase

Patients in the chronic phase died from various infectious complications and respiratory failure. In this phase, peripheral nerves exhibited an inflammatory neuropathy with a lymphocytic perineuritis leading to perineural fibrosis and secondary axonal degeneration. Muscle tissue showed interstitial inflammatory myopathy, followed by a neurogenic muscular atrophy as the disease progressed. The scleroderma-like skin lesions showed fibrosclerosis and vasculitis of the small arteries. The salivary glands also showed vasculitis and some interstitial inflammation that progressed towards interstitial fibrosis and parenchymal atrophy. The liver showed both portal area lesions and infiltration, as well as lobular changes, such as hepatocyte degeneration and infiltration. Some cholestasis was seen. Surprisingly, few changes were seen in the brain and kidneys. Six placentae from TOS patients showed no significant changes. Thus, the most prominent feature was the ubiquitous vascular lesion common to all the cases examined.

Chemical Studies of Oil Samples

Background and collection of samples

Initial analyses of case-related cooking oils showed that they contained mixtures of seed oils, mainly rapeseed oil. Samples were collected by food hygiene personnel or submitted by relatives of TOS patients or by other anxious consumers. Many of these samples contained aniline and fatty acid anilides, and some were traced to a packaging plant in Alcorcón near Madrid. Subsequent investigations showed that this company had obtained denatured rapeseed oil through the main importer in San Sebastián. The oil was then sent to two small refineries, one in Seville (60 tonnes) and one in Madrid (50 tonnes), for de-denaturation. The oil was refined in batches (each of 4.5 tonnes in Seville), and the possibility therefore exists that the refined product may have varied in quality and perhaps toxicity. The packaging company then mixed the refined oil (about 100 tonnes) with other oils and marketed the clandestine cooking oil as unlabelled olive oil in 5-litre plastic containers. According to the available records, the 100 tonnes of refined rapeseed oil were used and, with an average rapeseed oil content of some 40% in the final product, a total of 250 tonnes of clandestine cooking oil may have been marketed, partly through itinerant salesmen, partly through large-scale distributors. All suspect cooking oil was recalled as from the end of June 1981 and exchanged for pure olive oil by government order. About 3000 tonnes of oil were collected in this way, much of which was obviously not directly related to TOS. Owing to doubts about the exact identity of samples, some of the investigations during the emergency-like period following the outbreak of the TOS epidemic were inevitably misplaced. Furthermore, the lack of a reliable screening method meant that the toxicity of oil samples could not be established objectively.

Chemical composition

On the basis of considerable analytical work carried out at the National Centre for Food and Nutrition in Majadahonda, at the Institute of Fats and their Derivatives in Seville, and at institutions abroad, some conclusions may be drawn concerning the chemical composition of case-related oils. The oil consists mainly of rapeseed oil with some animal fat and grapeseed oil. Aniline is present only in traces, and fatty acid anilides usually occur in concentrations of 1000–2000 parts per million. Thus, although the toxicological significance of fatty acid anilides remains questionable, these compounds may nevertheless serve as indicators for toxic oil samples. No organochlorine or organophosphorus pesticides have been detected, and no heavy metals or other toxicants suspected. Certain organic compounds, such as chloropropanediol esters, have been found but, as with the fatty acid anilides, their toxic potential for causing TOS is not at all convincing.

Refining process
According to information released to the Working Group by the judicial authorities, the denatured rapeseed oil was refined in both Seville and Madrid according to standard procedures that are not especially directed at the removal of aniline. The refining consisted of four main steps: degumming, neutralization, bleaching and deodorization. The bleaching, in particular, led to a product with high cell culture toxicity in one experiment, and this finding could be related to the formation of aniline compounds, such as the benzoiminoquinone derivative of aniline. Studies at the Unilever Research Laboratorium in the Netherlands have shown that this complete refining procedure removed the free aniline but produced no fatty acid anilides, only higher molecular weight aniline derivatives of currently unknown identity and toxicity. Nevertheless, fatty acid anilides could be the result of spontaneous formation during storage before refining.

Experimental Toxicology

Considerable toxicological testing of oil samples has been carried out both in Spain and abroad. Ten different animal species have been used under various treatment regimens. Additional work is in progress. Nevertheless, the limitations imposed by the emergency affected the toxicological studies as it did the chemical studies of the oil samples. For example, when a British laboratory examined ten oil samples supplied from Spain, only three contained any anilides at all. Questions concerning the authenticity of such samples must be raised, and this problem obviously hampers the interpretation of the experimental results.

Test systems
In vivo studies have shown variable results. Perhaps the most promising species is the pig (or the mini pig), in which some pathological changes, perhaps related to TOS, have been caused by the oil. In the mouse, effects have been reported to include lipid peroxidation processes. In addition, some positive findings have resulted from work on the rabbit. These findings have not yet been reproduced in other laboratories, however, and their relevance to TOS has not been established. Other studies have rendered negative findings. The reasons for an absence of response may include the absence of toxins in the oil samples tested, the insensitivity of the animal model and, possibly, nutritional factors.

The independent replication of studies is imperative. Various *in vitro* test systems have been used and promising results have been obtained, in particular with the human fibroblast and the chick embryo systems.

The possibility of mycotoxins being a causative agent is suggested by the sporadic occurrence of rape poisoning. The two most likely candidates, trichothecenes and cytochalasins, are currently being assessed in oil samples, but preliminary findings have been negative.

Role of fatty acid anilides

Most attention has been paid to fatty acid anilides because of an early report of specific IgE antibodies in some patients. The acute toxicity of these compounds in mice is limited, with LD_{50} values (the dose that will kill 50% of the animals) in the g/kg range at least 10-fold higher than the LD_{50} values for aniline. However, glutathione-depleted mice showed a range of pathological responses after intraperitoneal injection of rapeseed oil with fatty acid anilides. In addition, toxic effects have been reported on the central nervous system of rabbits. Other studies using different experimental protocols have failed to produce any effect related to fatty acid anilides. Thus, the question regarding the possible role of these anilides in the pathogenesis of TOS remains open. In fact, other components of the oil not yet examined may well be better indicators of oil toxicity, and the cause of TOS could in principle be independent of fatty acid anilide concentrations.

2

Subgroup discussions

The participants divided into three subgroups to discuss and review detailed aspects of particular issues. The conclusions and recommendations that appear at the end of this report were proposed by these groups and accepted by the plenary session.

Epidemiology

One subgroup met with epidemiologists, public health officers and others who had conducted original studies or gathered information on the possible cause of the TOS epidemic. Data from the national system for case surveillance were examined. Specific information on the sources and distribution of suspect rapeseed oil was critically reviewed, as were data on causal hypotheses involving agents other than cooking oil. Results from several case-control studies were scrutinized, as was information on cases and clusters of cases.

Dr C. Heath was elected Chairman and Dr J. Rigau-Perez Rapporteur.

Surveillance data

Several population-based data files exist on TOS patients and members of their families or households.

1. Daily telephone notifications continue to be made by all hospitals to the Ministry of Health and Consumer Affairs of TOS cases admitted to hospital (without the personal identification of patients). Records of initial case admissions to hospital and readmissions from this source provide official incidence figures for Spain as a whole and for individual provinces.

2. Until October 1981, detailed information was sought by the Ministry of Health and Consumer Affairs on each TOS case notified by telephone. A total of 10 000 such case records was received, of which 7000 were entered into computer files.

3. In September 1981, a national census of all TOS cases was instituted on a continuing basis. This file now contains information on about

20 000 people. Information comes from the review of hospital and clinical records and from direct contacts with patients and their families. One major purpose of the census is to implement the national law that provides economic compensation to TOS patients in Spain, but the accuracy of all data items in the file has not been verified.

4. Separate registries of TOS cases are maintained by provincial authorities. The extent and accuracy of these files were not ascertained by the subgroup.

5. Between September 1981 and December 1982, personnel from the Ramón y Cajal Centre performed a nationwide survey of all the family members of 4000 TOS patients to assess the extent of undetected TOS illness. By similar efforts in other medical centres, a follow-up of 80% in an estimated population of 60 000 people nationwide was achieved. Although very few new cases were diagnosed, this data file contains systematic national information on people who were exposed in the family home.

Apart from the estimate of hospital admission rates and the search for new cases in families, these files have not yet been analysed in detail. Assuming that the material they contain can be collated and assembled in analysable form (if not *in toto,* then through a suitable sample of records), the subgroup suggested that these files could be used to answer certain important questions about the nature of this epidemic on a national scale and at the provincial level. Such questions include:

— the precise shape of the epidemic curve to determine if the abrupt fall in the onset of cases in June 1981 followed the Government's recall of oils (implying a causal effect) or preceded it (implying a decrease in toxin exposure from some other cause);

— whether acute illness early in the epidemic was more severe than acute illness later, implying a decline in the toxicity of the oil over time (by the dilution or decay of the toxin);

— whether or not the severity of acute illness (myalgia, eosinophilia) predicted the risk of chronic sequelae; and

— the frequency of familial illness according to case severity or time of illness (early or late in the epidemic).

Analytical investigations

Analytical epidemiological work (case-control or cohort studies) has been carried out on the risk factors associated with the occurrence of TOS and the risk of birth defects in children born to women with TOS or exposed to suspect oil. The subgroup reviewed data from nine separate case-control studies (see Annex 2) that compared patients with TOS, or their families, with controls (people without TOS, or their families) regarding the presence or absence of a wide range of personal or family characteristics or exposure considered to be potential risk factors for the development of TOS. Many of the risk factors studied involved items of food and the way they were prepared. The striking finding that was consistent in all these studies was a remarkably strong association between the development of TOS and the consumption of food oil purchased from itinerant vendors or salesmen.

Although most of the studies were conducted at the time of, or within a few days of, the Government's announcement declaring food oil to be the cause of TOS, the consistency and great strength of the epidemiological association are most unlikely to have been the result of bias because of this announcement. This judgement is confirmed by the fact that the same strong association was found in a study of 124 cases and 124 controls in a Madrid paediatric hospital in early June 1981, prior to the government announcement. The methods used in this study are described in Annex 1, and the results are discussed in Annex 2. A series of studies begun on 10 June in Navas del Marques (Avila province) found, in addition to the strong linkage with oil use, a dose–response pattern indicating greater oil consumption by affected patients than by their unaffected relatives and controls. Considering the urgent circumstances under which the remaining seven studies were performed, the subgroup believed that their collective findings about unmarked food oil as a risk factor in the development of TOS were a highly conclusive epidemiological observation. No strong or consistent evidence was found in these studies to suggest inhalation rather than ingestion as the route of oil exposure.

Case studies

Another category of epidemiological observation consisted of detailed information about particular cases with unusual features, or the particular circumstances of cases that gave insight into the possible nature of toxic exposure. Of special interest among such observations are ones that describe exposure to a single sample of oil at a particular time. Several such situations were described to the subgroup: cases among nuns at a convent in Madrid, and among residents of a pension in León; cases in a family receiving a single carafe of suspect oil from a gardener; the case of the Spanish wife of an American serviceman who visited her mother and acquired a single container of oil; and cases in one part of Soria province compared with cases in another part served by different oil salesmen. In each of these episodes estimates of latency, some quite precise, were remarkably consistent and suggested that the usual interval in adults from the first ingestion of oil to the first symptom was 7–10 days. It was further suggested, although no particular data were presented, that the latency in children was regularly somewhat shorter (3–4 days), perhaps a partial reflection of relative dose.

One striking case, however, seems at odds with these consistent observations. This involved a convent in Casarrubios del Monte in the province of Toledo, the reported birthplace of the brothers who owned the company (RAELCA) that is accused of treating and distributing the suspect oil. Many residents of this village were said to work for RAELCA delivering oil. Nuns at the convent allegedly received oil from RAELCA in early February 1981 but none thereafter. Some nuns fell ill in March and others as late as May, suggesting latencies of 1–3 months. Since the reliability of these particular observations cannot be effectively checked, their discrepancy can only be noted in contrast to what appears to be the more general latency as well as the accepted date of initial introduction of suspect oil.

In some cases, very small amounts of consumed oil seemed capable of inducing illness. This might suggest, although documentation is obviously difficult, that the toxicity of different oil aliquots may have varied greatly, perhaps according to the date of exposure (early as opposed to late in the epidemic).

Three cases occurred in Seville, and perhaps others in Granada, apparently as the result of the ingestion of oil obtained directly from the refinery in Seville, after the aniline de-denaturing and refining but before the mixture of rapeseed oil with oils from other sources. These cases are of particular interest because they suggest that the toxic agent may have been confined to rapeseed oil itself or to chemical manipulations involving such oil.

Other cases include the single occurrence of TOS in a baby breastfed by a mother with TOS. Although apparently an isolated event, this case is of obvious interest as it suggests transmission by maternal milk of whatever toxin is involved.

There appeared to be no evidence to support the suggestion that TOS or any illness related to it had occurred in domestic pets in Madrid or in pigs in Catalonia fed batches of the suspect oil.

Alternative hypotheses

The subgroup considered that the epidemiological evidence linking oil consumption with the occurrence of TOS was extraordinarily strong and consistent. By contrast, no convincing alternative hypothesis has been presented. The earliest hypothesis suggested that TOS was an infectious disease (see Annex 1). This possibility was thoroughly explored by laboratories in Spain and abroad, with completely negative results for a comprehensive list of infectious agents. In addition, certain pathological features of the illness seem unusual for infection, and there are good epidemiological grounds for discounting the idea. Although cases were concentrated in household groups (a setting quite compatible with shared food consumption), they did not aggregate in other traditional settings associated with the spread of infection (schools, dormitories, conventions, etc.) and did not appear among small infants. The subgroup reviewed two particular hypotheses other than that associating TOS with oil ingestion. One linked illness to the ingestion of tomatoes treated with certain pesticides, and the other proposed a relation to fungus infection or toxins produced by fungi associated with the grapeseed used to produce a common constituent of oil. Neither set of evidence seemed more than anecdotal. Appropriate epidemiological analyses testing the association of such risk factors with the occurrence of TOS have either not been done or were not at all convincing as presented to the subgroup. The pesticide-treated tomato hypothesis seemed particularly unreasonable as the epidemic of TOS has clearly ceased despite the alleged continued periodic use of the pesticides in question.

Clinical Observations and Pathology

Summaries of research carried out by specialists in a range of medical fields were made available to the Working Group through the Clinical Commission of the National Programme for the Toxic Syndrome, which is coordinating research and clinical management. Members of the Commission and researchers in charge of specific research projects met with the subgroup that was concentrating on clinical observations and pathology, to review and discuss the findings and the relationship to the possible pathogenesis and clinical course of TOS. A detailed review of the most important characteristics of TOS is given in Annex 3.

Professor M. Serrano-Rios was elected Chairman and Dr D. Geddes Rapporteur.

General features

Although the complete spectrum of TOS in its acute and chronic phases was a unique constellation of signs, symptoms and pathological findings, it did share some features with several other human disease conditions. In the acute phase, the presence of fever, myalgia, lymphadenopathy, noncardiogenic pulmonary oedema, eosinophilia and high IgE levels might suggest one of the many types of eosinophilic pneumonia. The pathology, however, was that of acute endothelial injury and interstitial oedema rather than pneumonitis; likewise, the dermal pathology was of endothelial injury with oedema and slight perivascular infiltrate.

Thus, this acute constellation of clinical and pathological changes in the absence of positive microbiological findings represented a new disease. There were similarities with the acute phase of graft-versus-host disease, a highly artificial situation without intensive long-term experience. Diffuse connective tissue disorders, such as scleroderma, dermatomyositis, or necrotizing vasculitis, do not demonstrate this acute intense syndrome. The mechanism of acute TOS seemed to be primarily toxic, with possible transient allergic features superimposed, and with little or no evidence of classical immunological mechanisms. Oedema was due to endothelial injury with a failure of selective permeability. Intravascular coagulation and failure of fibrinolysis leading to thrombosis were further signs of endothelial failure.

In the minority of subjects who progressed over months to develop the chronic syndrome there were similarities with several human disorders, most prominently scleroderma (systemic sclerosis), chronic graft-versus-host disease in patients receiving bone marrow transplantation, and various forms of vasculitis and toxic neuropathy.

The most compelling common denominator to explain the features of the chronic phase was the progression of the intimal lesion with proliferation of myointimal cells and the inflammation that led to a partial obliteration of the vessel lumen and organization of myofibroblasts. Autoantibodies were detected in some patients in the chronic phase, but no causal role has been established.

Pulmonary manifestations

The acute manifestations of TOS were predominantly seen in the lungs and skin. The acute syndrome was characterized by cough, fever, myalgia and a variety of skin rashes. Wheezes and râles were heard variably over the lungs, and chest radiographs showed interstitial and/or alveolar shadowing, sometimes with pleural effusion. Some patients died, most of them of respiratory failure, in the acute phase; the majority recovered within one or two weeks.

Pulmonary pathological findings from autopsy and a few transbronchial biopsies carried out in the acute phase showed the predominant involvement of the capillary endothelial cells, with minimal evidence of inflammation or eosinophilic infiltrate that could not be attributed to corticosteroid therapy. There was no conclusive functional or pathological evidence of airway involvement.

As the acute phase resolved, lung function tests, which had initially shown volume loss with impaired diffusion capacity for carbon monoxide (T_{CO}), improved; in the majority of patients, radiographs and lung function tests returned to normal in three months. About 20% of patients showed evidence of pulmonary hypertension, which resolved in all but 3%. Corticosteroid therapy may have assisted the resolution of the lung lesions. Pathological examination of the lungs in the chronic phase usually showed vasculitis of variable severity but no pulmonary fibrosis and only very exceptional cases of plexiform lesions of pulmonary hypertension.

Some patients continued to have abnormal T_{CO} measurements after initial impairment, and in one hospital a few patients (6 out of 42) showed a progressive decline in T_{CO} that cannot be explained in terms of malnutrition or general disability since the vital capacity remained normal.

Cardiac abnormalities have been detected on pathological examination but have not given rise to frequent or severe clinical problems.

Skin and endothelium

The skin demonstrated acute (exanthema and oedema) and chronic (fibrosis) phases that can be directly linked to the injury of the endothelium. It was unclear to the subgroup whether or not intervention could prevent the transition from the acute to the chronic phase. The proportion of patients in the acute phase who developed chronic skin changes was between 5% and 15%, a distinct and perhaps distinctive minority.

Nervous system

Neurological problems were the most serious cause of chronic disability. The clinical features were myalgia and muscle cramps, muscle weakness and wasting, sensory loss, and involuntary movements. Clear-cut central nervous system manifestations were less prominent.

A synthesis of clinical, physiological and pathological data suggests the following conclusions about site of damage and pathogenesis. Muscles were affected early by vascular and interstitial changes without much muscle fibre damage as judged by mild weakness, normal serum creatine phosphokinase, and histological appearances. Nerve involvement caused the severe wasting seen in the chronic stage and was characterized by an axonal neuropathy without significant myelin damage. The patterns included a diffuse sensorimotor neuropathy, mononeuritis of cutaneous nerves but not usually of mixed nerves, and a syndrome of profound motor involvement with relatively little sensory impairment. Pathologically, the nerves showed vascular inflammatory changes followed by profound interstitial fibrosis.

The evidence does not suggest an infective cause. Some features can be explained on a vascular basis: the interstitial changes in muscles and nerves, and the cutaneous mononeuritis. Most of the features are best explained by a direct toxic effect on neurons and their axons, and they resembled those of established toxic neuropathies in humans and other animals, although no analogy is exact. There were no features suggesting an autoimmune neuropathy or myopathy.

Changes in other organs

In the chronic phase of TOS, the sicca syndrome was common. The dryness of the mouth caused difficulty in mastication and swallowing and may have contributed to the development of severe, widespread dental caries.

About half the patients with a chronic clinical syndrome complained of dysphagia, and oesophageal studies of some of these patients have shown decreased peristalsis with abnormal oesophageal changes. Several factors may have contributed to this problem, including denervation, the sicca syndrome and structural changes in the oesophageal wall.

Extensive and reliable clinical data are available from families with TOS in which a pregnancy began around the time of the epidemic. Detailed cytogenetic studies have been done on a subgroup of parents and their offspring. The information available at present has not established any special damage to the mother, the fetus or the newborn child as a result of TOS.

Biochemical indications of abnormal liver function were frequent. In particular, signs of cholestasis were a common finding, as indicated by increased gamma-glutamyl transpeptidase and alkaline phosphatase and, in some cases, bilirubin. Signs of hepatic cytolysis, i.e. increased transaminases, were less frequent. At present, about 2000 patients, or about 10% of all cases, still exhibit such abnormalities. Clinical indications that the liver was affected occurred less often. Morphological changes, as assessed by a representative number of liver biopsies, seemed to be of a limited degree.

Toxicology

People who had conducted original research on oil samples and individual components of the oil had made summaries of their results available for review prior to the Working Group meeting. A detailed account of the chemical changes during the refining process is given in Annex 4. Detailed scrutiny of these results was then carried out by the subgroup on toxicology, with particular emphasis on the origin of oil samples, experimental protocol, the significance of possible artefacts and the reproducibility of results. Several members of the Group visited one of the research institutions in

Madrid to review the methods used and examine histology slides. Information on the refining of suspect rapeseed oil was released by the judicial authorities, and specific questions on the denaturation, transportation and illegal trade were answered by the authorities from the Irún customs office during the meeting.

Dr T.A. Connors and Professor A.M. Municio were elected Co-Chairmen, and Dr W.N. Aldridge and Dr R.L. Willson shared the duty of Rapporteur.

General research strategy

In order to define the toxic component(s) of rapeseed oil contaminated with aniline and with anilides and other substances produced during the refining process, studies should be carried out at the chemical, biochemical, cellular and whole animal level using: synthetic fatty acid anilides and other aniline derivatives identified as components of the toxic oil; rapeseed oil to which anilides and other material have been added; and selected case-related oils as defined below. This strategy for continued studies is based on a detailed review of past experience.

Chemical analysis

Since analysis by Spanish and foreign laboratories of selected samples has shown great variation in the composition of the oil, e.g. plant and animal sterols, and fatty acid anilides, and since no correlation has been found between TOS and known toxicants such as heavy metals, some mycotoxins, paraquat, insecticides and herbicides, no specific recommendations for analytical chemistry can be made until new evidence suggests that analysis for particular types of chemical would be useful. When truly toxic oils can be identified by a bioassay system, chemical fractionation and analysis can proceed.

Further experiments are needed to simulate the refining processes used at the time. Previous simulation experiments have been attempted but it is recommended that, with the full information now made available by the authorities, further attempts should be made to simulate as closely as possible the original refining procedure. Both chemical and toxicological studies should be carried out at each stage of the process.

Models of disease

The development of adequate model systems for TOS is of utmost importance. Without such systems, the identification of toxins and protective mechanisms, if they exist, cannot be carried out. In doing so, every aspect of experimentation is considered important. Attention must be paid to ensure that artefacts do not arise. Already, extremely important aspects of both animal experimentation and histopathological techniques in some experiments have been questioned. Such procedures can be improved in the future, and advice should be sought from qualified experts.

Ideally, a model system should reproduce all aspects of the disease. This may be impossible, however, and a number of *in vivo* and *in vitro* models may be necessary to piece together the various known components of the disease.

In vitro testing

Many *in vitro* procedures for assessing toxicity are available. Previous work on the oils has mainly used HeLa cells, human fibroblasts and the chick embryo. The subgroup agreed that HeLa cells were unsatisfactory. Experiments comparing toxic oils containing anilides and aniline derivatives with a variety of control oils have shown that the human fibroblast system is particularly sensitive to toxic oils and might be useful as part of a screening procedure. This work should be continued, but questions remain concerning the appropriate controls to be used and the role that other factors may play in the outcome of the assays. At a higher level of cellular organization, the chick embryo system appears promising and should be further evaluated.

In many cases there is doubt whether adequate controls were used. Neither a control system in a single laboratory nor an interlaboratory comparison has been set up to establish whether or not case-related oils can be distinguished from normal edible oils. Recognized procedures for setting up such blind trials are available for future use.

In vivo testing

The administration of many oil samples to baboons, monkeys, ducklings, guinea pigs and hamsters has given negative results. Using the rat, one laboratory reported lung damage, while there have been negative results from Spain and elsewhere. Using pigs, one centre reported clinical signs. Although there have been negative data on the mouse from many laboratories, one laboratory obtained clinical signs in mice treated with an oil sample collected soon after TOS was recognized. In another experiment, clinical signs were observed only when the mice were pretreated with diethylmaleate. On clinical grounds, the rabbit system appeared to be the most promising. The pathological changes claimed to be associated with the disease could not, however, be validated by independent examination of the histopathological preparations.

In spite of the efforts made in many countries, no animal model has been shown to be a reliable test system for toxic oil or anilides. Most systems give negative results while the positive results reported could be due to, for example, inadequate control of the experimental procedure or low-quality histopathology. Thus, any procedures yielding positive results should be repeated, using more rigorous methods.

Future research projects

Although there is no firm evidence as yet that fatty acid anilides are the toxin in the toxic edible oils, follow-up of any observations indicating biological activity of anilides should be encouraged. Biochemical changes have been observed, and while these may not be related to the disease process, they may offer clues as to the way they interact with biological systems. Among those changes observed after administration of samples of rapeseed oil (containing anilides) and synthetic anilides are modifications of lipid peroxidation, glutathione peroxidase (liver), glucose 6-phosphate dehydrogenase (lung), reduced glutathione (liver) and glucose 6-phosphatase and ATPase (liver and lung).

Two observations may lead to further significant research. It is now generally accepted that reduced glutathione acts as a scavenger of reactive electrophilic species. It is unknown whether the toxicity shown by oleilanilide is due to the parent compound or one of its metabolites. Depletion of the glutathione in mice by pretreatment with diethylmaleate increases the toxicity of oleilanilide, and the animals present a distinct clinical picture. The histological examination of tissues from these mice has been criticized, however, and has indicated deficiencies in the experimental protocol. Until these experiments are repeated, the significance of the findings cannot be assessed. When this reassessment has been made, other more specific methods of reducing glutathione should be examined and dose–response and structure–activity relationships established. In rats, administration of oleilanilide (30 mg/kg by gavage) leads to a marked loss of adipose tissue stores and to changes in the enzymic activity involved in lipid synthesis, particularly in lung and adipose tissue. It was reported to the subgroup that a similar depletion of these adipose tissue stores has been found after treatment of mini pigs. Since these two studies demonstrate biological activity of the anilides themselves, it is recommended that they be extended.

Evidence is emerging from experimental studies that vitamin E and selenium may exert some protective role. If indeed vitamin E and/or selenium do play a role in the disease process, their administration would most likely be effective before the toxic insult. Some attention should therefore be paid to the vitamin E (alphatocopherol) and selenium status of the population in Spain. Preliminary evidence has been presented that suggests that some people affected with TOS may be selenium-deficient. Such studies should now be extended using epidemiological sampling procedures, taking into account age, sex, diet, socioeconomic factors, human lymphocyte antigen types, etc. These factors may have a bearing on both the progression and the clinical sequelae of the disease.

Selection of case-related rapeseed oils for further study

The selection system for case-related oils in use up to the present has, in many cases, been unsatisfactory. Many laboratories in Spain and other countries have wasted much effort on samples that vary widely in composition and that in many cases contain no anilides. The subgroup recommended a new selection system.

The disease appears to have originated from the consumption of one or more batches of refined rapeseed oil denatured by aniline. The evidence that fatty acid anilides are the cause of the disease is not conclusive, but they may nevertheless be markers for toxic oil. The selection of oils for research work should be made according to the following criteria: they should be obtained from the homes of patients with TOS, and have a high content of rapeseed oil and anilides. Oil obtained from the refinery in Seville was 100% rapeseed oil and contained 1800 μg of anilides per g. All oils bought from itinerant salesmen are diluted with other fats and oils (up to 60%). It is proposed that the oils selected should contain no less than 40% rapeseed oil and 700μg of anilides per g.

For several oils fulfilling these criteria, chemical analysis and toxicity tests based on a standard experimental protocol should be carried out in laboratories in Spain and abroad.

3

Future action

The occurrence of this extraordinary disease in Spain has important implications for current and future responses with regard to food safety, contingency planning, epidemiological surveillance and research. Owing to the nature of this incident and the fact that the precise cause of TOS has so far eluded discovery, these implications may apply to other countries as well as Spain. These aspects were discussed in plenary session.

Post-emergency Response

The sudden occurrence of a severe epidemic calls for prompt responses. During the early phase of the outbreak, information on the probable source of the causal agent was dispersed as early as possible through the mass media, and an exchange of suspect oil samples was instituted only weeks later. Furthermore, a compensation plan for TOS victims has been developed. Unfortunately, at present, the various treatment regimens proposed have to be considered as purely experimental because the disease is incompletely understood and no particular treatment of chronic cases has proved successful so far. Future studies of potential treatment regimens must be conducted as controlled clinical trials to obtain the most valid information possible. In connection with the compensation plan, a registry has been compiled of all TOS cases in Spain. This registry is of unique value in the follow-up of the long-term effects of TOS. Such a follow-up may include both victims of the disease and household members not known to be afflicted with TOS. In the clinical management of TOS patients and in the continued medical and toxicological research on the cause and long-term significance of this disease, collaboration should be sought among institutions within and outside Spain. Coordination of these efforts should aim at increasing the efficiency of the work so that the maximum amount of information is gained.

The illegal manufacturing and distribution of contaminated rapeseed oil have dramatically illustrated the need for a more exacting food safety service at national and local levels. In addition, a coordinated system for contingency planning and emergency response is an obvious necessity. An efficient national programme on epidemiology is indispensable, and education and training in food safety and toxicology are an unavoidable requirement in the prevention of future incidents. The Working Group agreed that these considerations apply both to the specific TOS incident in Spain and to the wider preventive aspects of food-mediated toxicity in any country.

Government Support

In addressing the Working Group on the last day of the meeting, the Minister of Health and Consumer Affairs of Spain (Annex 5) supported the recommendations and conclusions reflected in the discussion and in the subgroup reports already presented. The Minister announced that the inspection team had been considerably extended and that regulations on edible vegetable oils had been passed in January 1983. He stressed that scientific conclusions, once adopted by the scientific community, should be respected by politicians, and that the Government of Spain intended to support, and not to interfere with, these scientific efforts. The conclusions and recommendations emanating from this meeting would help to initiate or strengthen a number of activities within the scope of work of the National Programme for the Toxic Syndrome. A new epidemiological commission would be formed to: review all existing epidemiological information; maintain active surveillance; verify the relationship between the consumption of oil from street vendors and the development of TOS; and determine from epidemiological data the relationship between the disease and possible toxic agents in the oil. The commission would also find substantial support in the recommendations concerning the establishment of biological test systems, the development of a simulated model for oil refining and the continuation of toxicological research. Such studies might need collaboration from research centres in other countries. The Minister conveyed his gratitude to the WHO Regional Director for Europe for the great speed and efficiency displayed in organizing the Working Group. On behalf of the Government, the Minister thanked WHO and the participants of the meeting and stressed that international collaboration was undoubtedly the best way to solve new health problems experienced in a complex socioeconomic context.

In closing the meeting, the Chairman thanked the national and international experts for being present and emphasized the Minister's words that politicians should respect scientific conclusions and not interfere with these complex questions. The Chairman expressed her gratitude, on behalf of the National Programme for the Toxic Syndrome, for the scientific results achieved and noted that the unfortunate victims of the disease would be equally grateful to the participants for their scientific contributions.

4

Conclusions and recommendations

Conclusions

Epidemiology

1. Nine separate case-control studies that compared patients with TOS, or their families, with controls (people without TOS, or their families) showed a remarkably strong and consistent association between the development of TOS and the consumption of food oil purchased from itinerant vendors or salesmen.

2. A series of studies begun on 10 June 1981 in Navas del Marques (Avila province) found, in addition to the strong linkage with oil use, a dose–response pattern indicating greater oil consumption by affected patients than by their unaffected relatives and controls.

3. No strong or consistent evidence was found in these studies to suggest inhalation rather than ingestion as the route of oil exposure.

4. Repeated clinical and epidemiological evidence suggests that the latency period between the ingestion of oil and the development of the first TOS symptoms was 7–10 days in adults.

5. From an epidemiological point of view, it is not yet clear whether aniline and aniline reaction products were present only in case-related oils, or whether de-denatured oil was in fact more widely distributed and consumed in Spain both before and during the epidemic and even in parts of the country unaffected by TOS.

6. In contrast to the findings with respect to food oils, no convincing alternative hypothesis has been put forward.

Clinical observations and pathology

7. TOS consisted of an acute and a chronic phase that showed features resembling those of well known disease entities, but the combined clinical picture and pathology findings are unique and suggest that this syndrome is new.

8. Characteristics of the acute phase included fever, eosinophilia, skin rash, pruritus, malaise, myalgia, arthralgia, dyspnoea, noncardiogenic pulmonary oedema and nonspecific gastrointestinal symptoms.

9. The mechanism of the acute phase of the syndrome seemed to be primarily toxic, with possible transient allergic features superimposed. The pathogenesis appeared to involve a systemic endothelial lesion with the most severe effects in the lungs.

10. The chronic phase, developing insidiously over a period of months, was characterized by peripheral neuropathy with muscle atrophy and deformity of the upper limbs, skin tautness of the scleroderma type, xerostomia and xerophthalmia (sicca syndrome), pulmonary hypertension and, less often, Raynaud's phenomenon, oesophageal hypomotility and the occurrence of autoantibodies.

11. The mechanism of the chronic phase has not been established. There were some features of toxicity and some of autoimmunity. The observed progression of the endothelial lesions suggests that the total array of chronic effects has yet to develop.

12. Less than 2% of the patients with TOS have died. The clinical course of most cases so far has been that of a slow, spontaneous resolution. In a small proportion of patients, the severe chronic changes described above have developed and, in a few patients, have not resolved. In addition, in a significant proportion of patients, an almost stable decrease of diffusion capacity of the lungs and/or increase of liver enzyme levels remain.

13. Corticosteroid therapy was beneficial and sometimes life-saving in the acute phase and subsequently speeded the improvement in lung function. There is no evidence that steroid therapy had either a beneficial or a harmful effect on the development and course of the neuromuscular syndrome. Although no harmful effect of steroid therapy has been detected, long-term treatment is not recommended.

14. Concerning other therapies, no overall benefit has been gained from any other drug treatment, and it is unrealistic to expect a specific antidote. Physical rehabilitation has been the most effective remedy for symptoms prescribed so far. Trials of other measures are still under way.

Toxicology

15. Owing to the emergency nature of the situation in 1981, proper organization of the collection of case-related oils and proper coordination of chemical and toxicological studies were not carried out.

16. Available evidence from chemical analyses and animal experiments is difficult to evaluate owing to the fact that different oils were examined in different laboratories, and uncertainty prevails as to whether or not truly case-related oil samples were examined.

17. Attempts to reproduce TOS in animal model systems have given many negative results. Moreover, the positive results obtained in one centre could not be reproduced in others. The reasons for these discrepancies may be due to the following factors in addition to the two mentioned above: the relevance of the animal models remains to be proved, the experimental design and processing of histological samples have, in some cases, been inadequate, insufficient attention has been paid to nutritional and other factors, and coordination between different groups of scientists has been insufficient.

18. Although an ideal model system should reproduce all aspects of the disease, a number of *in vivo* and *in vitro* models may be necessary to piece together a combined model system. In particular, promising preliminary results have been obtained with the human fibroblast system, chick embryo system and *in vivo* systems using the mouse and the rabbit. Nevertheless, all systems require validation.

19. The evidence that fatty acid anilides were the cause of the disease is still inconclusive, but they may nevertheless be useful markers for toxic oil.

20. Samples of aniline-denatured rapeseed oils kept by the customs authorities, samples of case-related oils kept at the National Centre of Food and Nutrition in Majadahonda, and those kept in connection with the National Programme for the Toxic Syndrome may become available for further study. In addition, technical details on the de-denaturation and refining operation at the refinery in Seville have just been released, thus perhaps making simulated toxic oil production possible.

General conclusion

21. It was the misfortune of the Spanish population that this extraordinary and unique disease made its appearance in their country. As long as the precise cause remains undiscovered, no assurance can be given that this type of disease will not occur again, perhaps in another country, for rapeseed oil and similar edible oils are widely used as items of diet throughout the world and, in their preparation and refining, they undergo various physical and chemical treatments that may modify their constitution. That is why, in particular, the elucidation of this incident in Spain demands the attention and efforts of other countries.

Recommendations

Epidemiology

1. Existing national and provincial TOS case-surveillance files should be verified, coordinated, and made accessible for active and continuing epidemiological analyses.

2. Existing case registries should be maintained on a continuing basis so that a periodic follow-up of TOS cases and their families can be made regarding possible health sequelae later.

3. To implement the first two recommendations and to enable adequate analysis of other epidemiological data, Spain should give high priority to developing a greatly strengthened national epidemiological programme. The availability of such a national resource would not only benefit studies of TOS but would also provide significant support for general activities in public health.

4. In view of the crucial importance and strength of the epidemiological evidence linking oil exposure to TOS development, it is strongly urged that all data in the nine case-control studies be promptly prepared for international scientific publication.

5. Although initial studies of birth defects in relation to TOS have shown no evidence of abnormal patterns, periodic reanalyses should be carried out, using national case files if possible, to take advantage of increasing numbers of observations and to exclude the possibility that evolving illness in patients with TOS may be accompanied by an altered risk of reproductive abnormality.

6. Clinical epidemiological data, particularly on specific kinds of oil and on latency periods, should be published in full where such data seem to have a firm basis and involve repeated observations.

7. A thorough reanalysis of all data on the time and place of distribution of food oils containing aniline or anilides should be carried out, thus enabling this difficult point to be resolved as far as possible.

8. As long as the exact toxin in the oil remains unidentified, all confiscated oil samples should be preserved in storage. Such samples should be clearly catalogued regarding their source, and their use as a foodstuff in the future should obviously be completely prohibited.

9. Any evidence suggesting the role of particular risk factors in TOS, as in any disease problem, needs to be fully presented for open scientific evaluation in the published scientific literature. If alternative hypotheses are to be considered, particularly in the face of convincing evidence regarding oil consumption, this useful and generally accepted procedure should be followed.

10. It could be of critical importance for more precise epidemiological and toxicological understanding of the epidemic and its cause if information now held by judicial authorities could be shared with scientific investigators.

Clinical observations and pathology

11. The organization of the follow-up of patients for the monitoring of the natural history of TOS and for future studies of clinical research should be concentrated on a small number of multidisciplinary units with central coordination. The medical care delivered to these patients, however,

whether in hospitals or in outpatient clinics, should be integrated with that for patients with other conditions.

12. A long-term follow-up programme should be set up to define the natural history of the disease and to detect and investigate deterioration. The follow-up groups should include: all patients with a persisting or progressing disorder of any organ system, which should be intensively investigated; the offspring of affected parents; patients who have made an apparently complete recovery; and exposed, but unaffected, individuals.

13. Collaboration in research and clinical management should be encouraged with centres outside Spain that have a special interest in related conditions or have special facilities for clinical investigation.

14. Any untried treatments should be considered entirely experimental. Such therapies should be given only as part of a properly planned and controlled clinical study in selected units.

15. The following general guidelines for further medical research are recommended: attention should be focused on endothelial damage and the repair of lesions; studies on both immunology and toxicity should be continued; and human lymphocyte antigen-typing of patients with both acute and chronic disease should be carried out on a sufficiently large scale for definite conclusions to be drawn.

Toxicology

16. A new coordinated approach is necessary to enable progress to be made in the possible identification of the toxic agent(s) in the oil and to elucidate the toxic mechanism and pathogenesis of TOS.

17. Oil samples for future studies should be selected on the basis of the following criteria: the sample should have originated from the home of a patient with TOS; the content of rapeseed oil should be at least 40%; and the content of anilides should be at least 700 μg/g.

18. Samples of oil collected at the time of the TOS outbreak are stored in the National Centre of Food and Nutrition in Majadahonda. After chemical analysis and initial screening on the Swiss mouse at Majadahonda, samples should be sent to other laboratories, both in Spain and abroad, for repeated testing according to agreed protocols.

19. A simulated procedure, based on that used at the refinery in Seville, should be used to produce samples of oil for chemical and toxicological characterization. Earlier agreements and recommendations in this respect should be implemented as soon as possible.

20. Research into the toxic properties of anilides and other aniline reaction products should be continued.

21. Mouse, rabbit, human fibroblast and chick embryo systems should be used for toxicity testing of the case-related oils as described above. At the moment, however, no particular bioassay system can be recommended.

22. An international steering group should be formed to evaluate the status of current research, to coordinate research activities, and to give guidance for future studies and the selection of oil samples for continued storage and further testing. It should also promote multicentre studies, develop joint protocols and arrange the peer review of experimental results.

23. In cooperation with the Government of Spain, WHO should explore sources of funds for international collaborative research into TOS. In addition, support should be sought from other international bodies because of the significance of this research with regard to human toxicology, defence mechanisms, and possible individual susceptibility related to nutritional factors.

24. The significance for health of food contamination and the particular catastrophic results of the toxic oil incident in Spain should be communicated in detail to government authorities abroad to emphasize the importance of food safety regulations, of the implementation of food inspection, and of strict enforcement practices.

General recommendations

25. The toxic oil syndrome, which has caused a tragic loss of life and serious illness, resulted from the illegal manufacture and distribution of an adulterated rapeseed oil sold for human consumption. It is important that consideration be given by the Spanish authorities to the need for more exacting food safety services at national and local levels, with adequate numbers of well trained inspectors supported by good legislation.

26. Expanded training programmes for Spanish personnel, if possible with international support, should be developed within the fields of toxicology, epidemiology and food safety.

27. In Spain, as in other countries, a well coordinated system is needed for contingency planning and emergency response to all types of chemical accident, to limit the severity of their effects. This system should be in accordance with the guidelines prepared by the WHO Regional Office for Europe under the International Programme on Chemical Safety.

28. The Working Group strongly supported the recommendations concerning epidemiology and clinical observations and pathology, and emphasized that they should be implemented without delay. There is an urgent need for further toxicological research in accordance with the recommendations. This work should be carefully planned and coordinated. This task might well be entrusted to a small group of individual experts from Spain and other countries.

29. The further activities recommended by the Working Group will require adequate funding. It is important that a programme to solve the problem of TOS should not be constrained by lack of commitment and material resources. The commitment should not be confined to Spain, because the possibility of another catastrophe of this kind elsewhere cannot be dismissed.

Annex 1

Discovery of toxic oil as the cause of the epidemic

J.M. Tabuenca Oliver

Onset of the epidemic

On 1 May 1981, an 8-year-old boy, one of eight members of a family from Torrejón de Ardoz, died from acute respiratory insufficiency. Six members of the family eventually fell ill with a similar clinical picture, unknown up to that time. On 4 May, the report on several cases of the new disease reached the Directorate General of Public Health, and a group of medical technicians carried out an investigation in Torrejón and visited patients in the del Rey and La Paz hospitals. At the Ramón y Cajal Centre, *Legionella gormanii* was isolated from a patient. On 6 May, the Office of the Secretariat of State for Health set up microbiological, clinical and epidemiological working groups. On 9 May, the Clinical Commission was established and it at once called a meeting of the directors of Madrid hospitals to report on the existence of an epidemic outbreak that could be caused by *Legionella* spp. At that meeting, the 23 cases reported up to that time were reviewed, the majority of them being adults, and the family occurrence was noted. The Commission, with the collaboration of pneumologists, had classified the illness as an atypical pneumonia, perhaps caused by *Mycoplasma* spp., a disease that would respond very rapidly to treatment with erythromycin, and this treatment was therefore recommended for all patients. The meeting also concluded that it was of the greatest importance for the diagnosis to verify the presence of a very variable interstitial pneumonia in the patient. Later, the Commission announced the hospitals to which patients should be sent. On the same day, different working groups were formed (paediatrics, pneumology, etc.) and a permanent secretariat was established for round-the-clock information. By 11 May, 150–200 new cases a day were being recorded, not only in the Madrid province, but also in the provinces of Avila and Segovia, and from 13 to 16 May and onwards in Valladolid, Palencia, Salamanca, León, Soria, Burgos, Zamora, Toledo and Santander. From that time, the number of new cases grew exponentially, and by 6 June, 2000 patients had been admitted to hospital in Madrid and 600 in the provinces. The number of emergency cases seen in hospitals had dramatically increased, with 341 admissions a day.

After 120 days of the epidemic, the number of deaths had risen to 100, and 12 000 patients had been in hospital. By December 1982, the number of cases recorded was 20 178. There were 85 patients still in hospital at that time, 10 of them in intensive care units. A total of 336 deaths had occurred, and 2250 patients were undergoing rehabilitation.

Initial studies at Niño Jesús Hospital

The explosive outbreak of the epidemic threatened to overflow the hospitals, and it was decided to send affected children to Niño Jesús Hospital from 12 May. Detailed studies of the epidemic in the child population began on this date. The first objective was to analyse, evaluate and classify the clinical picture and the complementary data; the following conclusions were immediately reached.

1. The illness was a previously unknown entity in children. The exanthema was similar in nature to toxico-allergic exanthemas by its distribution, colour, morphology, pruritus and evolution.

2. All the symptoms, which lasted an average of 1.6–3.7 days, of drowsiness, insomnia, slow mental reactions, irritability, photophobia, conjunctivitis, enanthema and flushed cheeks (deep red with a bluish hue) pointed in the same direction.

3. The chest X-ray corresponded to a severe pulmonary oedema and not to a picture of atypical pneumonia. In addition, this phenomenon was not constant but varied widely so that its absence could not exclude the diagnosis of the case, as originally thought.

4. Total disappearance of the sometimes massive interstitial pneumonia and the fever, after 3–7 days, did not correspond to the known evolution of atypical pneumonia, even after treatment with erythromycin.

5. The existing hepatosplenomegaly and the generalized ganglionic infarctions, together with all the foregoing, were interpreted as the expression of a systemic disease.

6. The considerable eosinophilia could not be attributed to any known paediatric nosological entity.

7. On the basis of these considerations, this illness was designated a toxic-allergic syndrome from 12 May, without reference to any specific causal agent.

Search for the cause of the toxic-allergic syndrome

At that time, with the diagnosis corresponding to an intoxication rather than to an infection, the following plan was put forward.

— A wide survey was to be carried out to identify possible microbiological and toxic agents by respiratory, digestive and dermal routes;

— different random and comparable patient groups were to be established and treated with antibiotics, antihistamines, corticoids, and symptomatic medication;

— a specially supervised placebo control group was to be set up;

— the toxicological literature was to be reviewed; and

— a laboratory was to be identified with specialized personnel and instrumentation for studies of selected agents or compounds.

A few days after these guidelines had been decided, the evolution of the disease in the different treatment and control groups was similar, with the exception of the group treated with steroids. This treatment caused a normalization of eosinophil numbers that increased again when the treatment stopped.

On 13 May, the National Microbiology Centre at Majadahonda and La Paz Hospital announced that mycoplasmata had been found in some autopsies. At the same time, the director of a hospital for infectious diseases attributed the epidemic to spring onions attacked by parasites, to rickettsia and later to strawberries, vegetables, asparagus and chicken. This statement caused considerable economic losses in agricultural sectors. Later still, he blamed the disease on dogs, cats, birds, etc. and this suspicion caused the extermination of many pets which drew protests from the animal protection societies. Rumours attributed the disease to organisms produced for bacteriological warfare and to radiation from the American military base at Torrejón. These rumours and allegations caused confusion and collective panic, and many terrified families fled from the epidemic areas.

In the survey at Niño Jesús Hospital, a questionnaire dealt with alimentary intake, in particular the following: organoleptic characteristics; frequency of consumption; fresh food and manner of preparation; preserved food; metal, cardboard, glass, and china in contact with food; home-preserved, bulk food; meals taken at home and outside; meat, fish, vegetables, carbohydrates, pastas, eggs, potatoes; fruit (type, with or without skin); jams; sausages; dairy products such as milk (whole, skimmed, sterilized, pasteurized, etc.), cheeses, yogurts, cottage cheese, butter, puddings, cream, junket, custards; bakery food such as bread, fritters, confectionery products, buns, pastries, cakes; chocolates; instant foods such as soup, puddings, purées; sauces and condiments; water; salt; vinegar; oil; appetizers such as potato crisps, bacon twists, olives, almonds, peanuts; infusions, juices, soft drinks, milk shakes; wine and spirits. In addition, each individual could include data that were thought to be of particular interest for the survey.

Among the epidemiological phenomena noted, the following facts attracted attention. The epidemic was explosive, spread rapidly and occurred mainly in the industrial belt of Madrid. Cases were not seen, however, in underprivileged groups, such as gypsies, and no aggregations were seen in hospitals, schools or barracks. The family connection between patients and the frequent readmissions of patients to hospital were notable. Further, no children under six months old were affected. The dissemination of the epidemic corresponded to a commercial distribution network by road rather than to the morphology of any other known type of infectious disease epidemic.

Confusion concerning possible cause

Around 20 May, considerable chaos occurred in the media. The most absurd hypotheses were spread about the possible causal agents, and this confusion only increased the anxiety of the population. On 21 May, however, the Minister of Health and Consumer Affairs, backed by his technical aides and in accordance with the official investigation, announced on television that the cause was a mycoplasma, and on 22 May he said that there was not a single datum in favour of transmission by the digestive tract.

On 21 May, after explaining the hypothesis and observations concerning a possible food contaminant, the author obtained the collaboration of the laboratories of the Institute of Hygiene and Safety at Work to determine heavy metals in specimens from patients, although the disease did not correspond to any typical clinical picture of metal intoxication. At the same time, evaluation of cholinesterase was initiated at Niño Jesús Hospital.

On 22 May, a foreign news agency reported that a stockpile of bacteriological weapons was kept at Torrejón de Ardoz, and that the epidemic had been caused by the escape of a virus or by a radioactive emission from bombs stored there. Maps were therefore made of the delivery routes for F-16 aircraft parts; coincidentally, these routes later turned out to be the ones used by the delivery trucks and mules that carried the toxic oil.

A few days later, the following were excluded as causal agents: viruses, mycoplasmata, bacteria, parasites and, among the intoxicants, heavy metals and organochlorine and organophosphorus insecticides. All these substances have a different clinical picture and were not indicated by the laboratory studies. On 27 May, an official report was made of all this information.

Collaboration was then established with the Central Customs Laboratories, which are directed by Professor Hernandez Bolanos, a laboratory expert in the detection of unsuspected foreign substances in imported and exported goods. Naturally, the detection of a possible unknown toxic substance, without any guideline for examining the biological specimens from patients, was going to prove a very difficult and slow process. At that time, the pressures, anguish and social panic were dramatic even among physicians. The most widely accepted hypothesis continued to be that the responsible agent was a mycoplasma, and trichinosis had begun to be considered as a second possibility.

Intoxication emerges as likely cause

For all the above reasons, and because it was now clear that a national catastrophe was inevitable, the author announced in a television interview on 1 June that according to his work, the epidemic was not caused by any microbiological agent, but by food poisoning, and that his work, already quite advanced, was continuing to explore this possibility. A few days earlier, the director of a Madrid hospital had been dismissed by the Ministry of Health and Consumer Affairs for making similar statements that were not in agreement with the official interpretation of the possible cause. A television station nevertheless broadcast the announcement in case anybody else working along the same lines discovered the responsible agent. Fortunately, this view was well accepted by the Ministry.

From an epidemiological viewpoint, it was especially interesting to examine small children, who spend most of their time at home and have a controlled and constant food intake, but who were nevertheless mostly unaffected by the epidemic. Another surprising phenomenon was that many patients who had been in hospital and been discharged in a much improved condition, later suffered a relapse and had to be readmitted to hospital, sometimes seriously ill. We began to examine what they had done in their homes, and interest focused on those who had had a shorter stay at home before the relapse, i.e. fewer than 7 days. Finally, the households with a large proportion of sick family members, as well as closed communities with high attack rates, were also of particular interest. In view of the dramatic situation and some negative response to the survey, the author decided to make the inquiries personally, following the criteria mentioned, in order to analyse each of the relevant details relating to the possible causal agents.

After the disease had been linked to food oil, a second food survey was carried out, using the following questions.

1. Does the patient eat tarts, buns, pastries, butter rolls, cakes?

2. Type of bread eaten and where it comes from?

3. Does the patient eat fried potatoes, popcorn, *ganchitos*? Where are they bought?

4. Does the patient go to nursery school or school? If so, give name and address. Dayboarder? Other school mates with atypical pneumonia?

5. Has the patient taken meals in the home of anyone with atypical pneumonia?

6. Does the patient often take appetizers in bars or cafes? What type of food does he usually take in these establishments?

7. Does the patient mix food oil?

8. What is the brand name of the oil he consumes? Where is it bought?

9. Are potato chips made at home or bought in a bag?

10. Is frying oil re-used? How many times?

11. Is refried oil added to purée?

12. Are pork fats, butter or margarine used for anything?

13. Are many precooked dishes used?

14. Has the patient attended family parties at which meals were eaten?

15. Has the patient attended neighbourhood festivities, *verbenas,* or similar events? What did he eat?

16. Does the patient eat mayonnaise, sauces or creams ready prepared? Brand? Where bought?

17. Does the patient eat doughnuts? Where bought?

18. Does the patient eat filled buns? Brand? Where bought?

Clandestine oil as causal factor

When this method was applied, it did not take long to detect a clandestine olive oil sold by street vendors in 5-litre plastic containers at 105 pesetas a litre, well below the usual market price for this type of oil. In the first days of June, the possibility of toxic compounds was raised by the epidemiological analyses. In the survey, details were gathered on the organoleptic characteristics of each of the possible food items, as well as their place of origin, place of purchase, trademark and container description. Thus, the consumption of clandestine oil was found and samples were obtained for analysis. A total of 97% of patients had consumed this oil, while of the unaffected people living in similar areas, only 6.4% had consumed it.

Chemical analyses showed that the oil consisted of a variable mixture of oils: sunflower and grapeseed oil, animal fats, and rapeseed oil originally denatured with 2% aniline and intended for industrial use. The food oil contained 50 ppm of aniline and some 1500 ppm of fatty acid anilides originating from the denatured rapeseed oil.

These facts were reported to the health authorities as well as verbally to the Minister of Health and Consumer Affairs; on 9 June, the author officially and personally informed the Minister who, in response to the results of the analyses, ordered on 10 June that the population of Spain should be told of the serious risk involved in consuming this oil. On the same day, all the media announced the finding of the toxic oil. From that time, hospitals and provincial health authorities started to focus on clandestine oil as a causal factor. In retrospect, the lack of supporting evidence apart from the studies at Niño Jesús Hospital is unfortunate.

Containers with oil and lists of suppliers and vendors were submitted to the Ministry of Health and Consumer Affairs and the Ministry of Agriculture. Oil for detailed chemical analyses then began to arrive in Majadahonda. At that time, the following agents in the food oil had already been excluded:

— mixtures with mineral oil, such as those that have occurred in Morocco and Jamaica with contaminants of the orthocresolphosphate type;

— aniline, nitrobenzene, acetylanilide and other compounds causing methaemoglobinaemia, because they were not present in sufficient doses in the oils analysed and because methaemoglobinaemia was not found in the patients;

— erucic acid, because its concentration was lower than 0.5%;

— heavy metals, because they were undetectable in the oil, they only occurred in trace amounts in biological samples from patients, and because the associated clinical pictures did not appear like the toxic-allergic syndrome;

— mycotoxins of the aflatoxin type, because they were not detected in the oil;

— organophosphorus insecticides (rejected clinically because cholinesterase was normal in the patients); chlorinated insecticides (rejected because the clinical picture was very different); and paraquat (excluded because it is water soluble, and the clinical picture of its intoxication differs);

— maleic anhydride, responsible for the intoxication caused by margarine in an epidemic in the Netherlands (no illegal use of this compound in the chemical extraction of fats from crude oils was detected);

— cutting oils, after analysis of the oil and by its odour, and tung oil (*Aleurites fordii*), because UV absorption was not high;

— leaching of toxic substances from the plastic containers, because they varied and came from different origins, and because analytical checks on the oil were negative;

— chloride and nickel, because of their variable occurrence, mostly only in trace concentrations too small to be of toxic significance;

— a combination of two agents, such as toxic oil and mycoplasma infection, because of the minimal incidence of the infection; and

— mycotoxins caused by fungi in the grapeseed.

Morbidity caused by the epidemic

As soon as the causal agent was known and as eosinophilia was an important indicator, the author suggested that a check should be made of the difference between the incidence of eosinophilia in the months of May and June of the year before the outbreak of the epidemic and the current level of eosinophils in asymptomatics. The purpose of this comparison was to get an approximate and overall impression of the extent of the epidemic. This work showed that there were approximately 10 times more asymptomatic people at risk than there were registered cases.

Despite the warnings concerning clandestine oil, a large proportion of the population was ignoring the risk because the media had broadcast all kinds of causal hypotheses. This fact was reported to the Ministry of Health and Consumer Affairs. On 26 June, in the television programme *La clave,* which has one of the largest viewing audiences, the guests included the Minister of Health and Consumer Affairs, an epidemiologist from the Centers for Disease Control in Atlanta, Georgia, a representative of WHO, the President of the Consumers' Association, the Director of the National Virology Centre, the Director of the Bacteriology and Virology Centre at the Ramón y Cajal Centre in Madrid, and the author. Taking advantage of the opportunity provided by this discussion, the author asked the Minister whether he would be willing to withdraw all toxic oil and exchange it at government expense with pure olive oil, because families with modest incomes were concerned. The Minister accepted the suggestion. The exchange operation began on 30 June, at which date the tremendous number of patients and deaths decreased drastically.

Annex 2

Summary of case-control studies and case or cluster investigations

J.G. Rigau-Perez

The subgroup on epidemiology reviewed the development of the TOS epidemic in May and June 1981 and the design of the investigations that showed an association between the illness and the consumption of illegally marketed cooking oil. The present paper outlines the two major groups of studies that were available for review: case-control studies in which the prevalence of many exposure factors was compared in cases and controls, and case or cluster investigations in which the peculiar circumstances of exposure for each case helped define the consequent risk.

Case-control studies

On 10 June 1981, the media announced the finding of an association between TOS and the consumption of illegally marketed oil. In studies performed after that date, respondents were aware of the reason for inquiries about oil consumption. The case-control studies were therefore considered in two groups.

Studies undertaken before 10 June 1981

The food ingestion histories of approximately 30 patients with TOS interviewed from 1 to 4 June 1981 were similar regarding oil consumption. From 4 to 8 June 1981, additional patients with TOS were interviewed; controls for all cases were interviewed in the surgical wards. Both groups (124 cases and 124 controls) had comparable socioeconomic status as all came from the hospital's catchment area. All the patients with TOS reported the consumption of illegally marketed cooking oil, defined as presumed olive oil sold in unlabelled, 5-litre plastic containers. Only 6.4% of the controls reported the use of this type of oil (*1*).[a]

Although other food ingestion surveys carried out before 10 June found that illegally marketed oil was a common factor among patients with TOS, none of them seems to have included interviews of controls (*2*).

[a] The methods of this study are described in Annex 1.

Studies undertaken after 10 June 1981

In a survey performed on 11 June, 27 case families, 54 size-matched and 54 randomly chosen comparison families were interviewed. All the case families had consumed illegally marketed cooking oil, defined as cooking oil in unlabelled, 5-litre or larger containers purchased from itinerant salesmen. By contrast, only 13 of the size-matched and 17 of the randomly chosen families had purchased this oil. Within the case families, the estimated amount of oil consumed per person was positively correlated with illness. A subsequent study on 9 July found that the major difference between the case and control families who had consumed the oil was whether the oil was purchased from a particular itinerant salesman. In April and May 1981, 24 out of 32 case families had bought their oil from this salesman (identified by his appearance, vehicle and streetcry) but only 5 out of the 23 control families had done so (*3*).

Investigations were conducted by personnel from the Ministry of Health and Consumer Affairs. In a survey performed on 15–22 June by Dr Catalá and co-workers in Chozas de Abajo, León, 19 case families, 19 families matched for size, sex ratio and age, and 19 randomly chosen comparison families were interviewed. All respondents (19/19 case families and 15/19 random control families) had purchased illegally marketed oil, as defined above. By contrast, 9 out of the 19 case families and 3 out of the 15 random control families had purchased the oil from specific vendors in the last two weeks of April 1981.

In another survey, performed on 19 June, by personnel from the Ministry of Health and Consumer Affairs, all the families in Cerezo de Arriba, Segovia, were interviewed. Of 13 case families, all had consumed illegally marketed cooking oil, while only 25 out of 44 healthy families had consumed it (*4*).

Investigations were also conducted by provincial health personnel in small rural locations using the same questionnaire as was used in León by the Ministry of Health and Consumer Affairs staff. Ten case families and ten control families were interviewed in San Cristóbal de Entreviñas, Zamora. All the case families reported consumption of illegally marketed cooking oil, while 3 out of the 10 control families had consumed it. All 44 families in Bocigas de Perales, Soria, were interviewed: all 11 case families but none of 33 controls had used the oil. In Arconada, Palencia, all 18 case families and 12 out of 21 control families had consumed the illegally marketed cooking oil.

Finally, investigations were conducted by preventive health personnel from Madrid medical centres. In a survey performed on 17 and 18 June, 48 families of patients from Pozuelo de Alarcón (Madrid) admitted to Puerta de Hierro Clinic with a diagnosis of TOS and 96 neighbourhood control families were interviewed. It was found that 42 of the case families and 32 of the controls had bought oil from itinerant salesmen. Because the purchase of products from itinerant salesmen was significantly more common among people with TOS than among controls, a reanalysis of the data was performed. Considering only the 43 case families and 58 control families that had reported purchasing products from itinerant salesmen, 41 case families had purchased oil compared with 32 control families (*5,6*). In a comparison of 20 families of patients from Colmenar Viejo (Madrid) admitted to the Ramón y Cajal Centre with a diagnosis of TOS and 20 neighbourhood control families, 16 case families and 6 control families reported exposure to illegally marketed cooking oil (*7*).

Case or cluster investigations

Santa Cruz Convent. In this community of 23 nuns cloistered in Casarrubios del Monte, Toledo, 20 cases of TOS, including one death, were reported. The convent purchased 75 litres of "olive oil" and 75 litres of "sunflower oil" from RAELCA in the first 10 days of February 1981, not buying any more oil afterwards. In March and April, several nuns fell ill, complaining of tiredness, but the first case with respiratory symptoms ("feeling of suffocation") did not appear until the end of May. The healthy nuns reported a lower consumption of salads, no use of oil as a salad dressing, and a higher consumption of milk than the nuns who fell ill. The town of Casarrubios is the birthplace of the Ferrero brothers, the owners of RAELCA, and 41 of the villagers allegedly made their living selling their unlabelled oil. Surprisingly, only six villagers (from four different families) developed TOS (*8*).

Convents located in Madrid. The custom in the convent at Calle Fuencarral 97 is to use soybean oil for most cooking purposes and olive oil for salads or special diets. In early May, two 5-litre containers of JAB oil were purchased at a special price from the convent's usual supplier, a grocery store on Calle Corredera. On 15 May, 23 novices, 2 sisters, a priest, and a teacher went to the country on a religious retreat and used the JAB oil for salads and sauces. On 23 May, some novices developed dyspnoea and by 25 May, all but 4 of the 27 participants were ill. The four exceptions were the priest, who ate very little, and three novices, who drank more milk than the others. The oil in the other 5-litre container was used very sparingly by the ten nuns remaining in Madrid and was used up mostly by the novices on their return to town. Only one of the ten that remained in Madrid developed TOS; another one died with multiple pains, but the diagnosis of TOS was not suspected owing to her age (90). None of the 56 boarders in the convent, who ate the same meals but did not use the JAB oil, developed TOS (*9*).

The 43 nuns in the convent at Calle Fuencarral 99 purchased three or four containers of JAB oil, at an unspecified date, to use for all cooking purposes. All became sick, except for a nun who was away from 18 May to 3 June. As in the other convent, none of the 60–80 boarders developed illness, and they shared the same food as the nuns, except the JAB oil for salads (*9*).

Cases related to the ITH refinery in Seville. Two family clusters (of three cases each) can be traced to the ingestion of "refined" rapeseed oil, undiluted with any other vegetable or animal fats. Both heads of household worked at the ITH refinery and brought home a container of unmixed rapeseed oil from RAELCA, after it had been "refined" at ITH. The oil was analysed at the Institute for Fats and their Derivatives in Seville (*10*).

Cases at a pension. Two guests started eating at the Pension La Asturiana, in Sahagún de Campos, León, on 4 May, and developed symptoms on 16 and 22 May, respectively.

Other cases. Three other cases have been reported. The wife of an American serviceman first bought this type of oil on 27 April, and fell ill 10 days later. A Bilbao resident ate meals prepared with illegally marketed oil in Escobar de Campos on 1–3 May and 15–17 May, and developed symptoms on 17 May. Finally, a woman moved to her sister's house on 3 May, where she ate foods prepared with illegally marketed oil. She was admitted to hospital on 16 May for cardiac decompensation, but a diagnosis of TOS was made on 20 May.

Conclusions

The members of the subgroup on epidemiology concluded that the repeated findings in separate case-control studies of unlabelled food oil as a risk factor for the development of TOS are a highly conclusive epidemiological observation. The cases related to unmixed, refined rapeseed oil from the ITH refinery in Seville suggest that the toxic agent is not related to the other substances used to dilute the rapeseed oil before distribution. The estimates of a latency period were remarkably consistent among the different case and cluster investigations, and suggest that in adults the usual interval from the first ingestion of oil to the onset of symptoms was in the range of 1–2 weeks. The exception to this is the convent in Casarrubios del Monte, where the latency period seems to have been 1–3 months. With the information available, it was impossible to account for this discrepancy.

References

1. **Casado Flores, J. et al.** Encuesta alimentación a niños con síndrome tóxico [Food survey of children with toxic syndrome]. *In: Simposium Nacional "Síndrome Tóxico" [National Symposium on the Toxic Syndrome], Madrid, 11–12 June 1982.* Madrid, Ministry of Health and Consumer Affairs, 1982, pp. 224–225.
2. *Informe del gobierno sobre actuaciones de la administración del Estado en relación con la enfermedad asociada con el consumo de aceite tóxico* [Government report about the State's administrative actions in relation to the illness associated with the consumption of toxic oil]. Madrid, Ministry of Public Health and Social Security, 1981, pp. 54–55.
3. **Rigau-Perez, J.G. et al.** Estudios epidemiológicos sobre el síndrome tóxico en Navas del Marques (Avila) [Epidemiological studies on the toxic syndrome in Navas del Marques (Avila)]. *In: Simposium Nacional "Síndrome Tóxico" [National Symposium on the Toxic Syndrome], Madrid, 11–12 June 1982.* Madrid, Ministry of Health and Consumer Affairs, 1982, pp. 217–219.

4. **Gil, E.** *Investigación epidemiológica sobre la neumonía atípica en la localidad segoviana de Cerezo de Arriba* [Epidemiological investigations of atypical pneumonia in the Segovian town of Cerezo de Arriba]. Madrid, Ministry of Public Health and Social Security, 1981 (unpublished report).
5. **Andres, J. et al.** *Informe preliminar de la investigación epidemiológica sobre la llamada "neumonía atípica" en Pozuelo de Alarcón* [Preliminary report of the epidemiological investigations on the so-called "atypical pneumonia" in Pozuelo de Alarcón]. Madrid, Unit of Preventive Medicine, Puerto de Hierro Clinic, 1981 (unpublished report).
6. **Andres, J. et al.** Epidemiología causal del síndrome tóxico [Epidemiological causes of the toxic syndrome]. *In: Simposium Nacional "Síndrome Tóxico" [National Symposium on the Toxic Syndrome], Madrid, 11–12 June 1982.* Madrid, Ministry of Health and Consumer Affairs, 1982, pp. 178–180.
7. **Lopez Abente, G. & Yuste Grijalba, J.** *Resultado del estudio de casos-control, Colmenar Viejo* [Results of the case-control study at Colmenar Viejo]. Madrid, Department of Preventive Medicine, Ramón y Cajal Centre, 1981 (unpublished report).
8. **Catalá Villanueva, F.X.** *Summary of the questioning made at the convent of "Santa Cruz" of Casarrubios del Monte, Toledo, 20 January 1982.* Madrid, Ministry of Health and Consumer Affairs, 1982 (unpublished report).
9. *Report on the visit to the convents located on No. 97 and 99 Fuencarral Street.* Madrid, Clinical Commission of the National Programme for the Toxic Syndrome, 1981 (unpublished report).
10. *ITH, Seville.* Madrid, Clinical Commission of the National Programme for the Toxic Syndrome, 1983 (unpublished report).

Annex 3

Clinical and pathological features of TOS

M. Serrano-Rios and V. Faro

The impact of TOS on the Spanish population has been considerable. The historical background and the epidemiological aspects have been well described elsewhere (*1–3*) and are beyond the scope of this paper. By December 1982 (*4*), it was estimated that 20 178 people had been affected by TOS. This figure was essentially unmodified by March 1983 (20 195, 60% of the patients being female). Of these more than 20 000 patients, 12 000 required hospital admission and 339 had died by May 1983. As of June 1983, it was estimated that 80% of the total population of patients could be considered clinically and biochemically "free of the disease", but 2000 still required regular physiotherapy owing to neurological sequelae (*4*). In June 1983, only five patients remained in intensive care units because of respiratory failure secondary to neurogenic muscle atrophy. Females were affected more often than males (1.6 : 1), particularly in the 30- to 40-year age range, and this sexual skewing was even more striking as TOS advanced into the multisystemic, clinically severe late phase.

Natural history: clinical phases

The natural history of TOS is now known in considerable detail, and several excellent clinical descriptions based on prolonged (from months up to two years) follow-up of hundreds of patients are available (*1,5,6*). For the purposes of clarity, the evolution of TOS has been artificially divided into two main phases: acute, comprising the two-month period of May and June 1981, and chronic, starting in July/August 1981 and continuing up to the present. In practice, patients suffering the whole evolutionary potential of TOS showed a continuum of slowly changing clinical syndromes. While the total number of affected people is well defined, it has been virtually impossible to establish the relative proportions of those suffering one only or both phases of TOS. It seems, however, that the majority of people affected initially were cured during the first four-month period, with some 15–18% of the total patient population entering the chronic phase of the disease. It has also proved difficult to define the predictor factor, or factors, for the transition of individual patients into the chronic phase. A possible genetic predisposition suggested by some human lymphocyte antigen studies needs further confirmation.

Acute phase: general features

During the acute phase, TOS typically appeared as a complex combination of severe respiratory symptoms (cough, dyspnoea) with striking chest X-ray changes most often showing diffuse interstitial patterns suggesting non-cardiogenic pulmonary oedema. Also present were constitutional complaints of variable severity (fever, malaise, asthenia, anorexia), nonspecific gastrointestinal symptoms (nausea, vomiting, diarrhoea, abdominal pain), skin rashes and pruritus, myalgias and arthralgias. Pulmonary râles, mostly at the lung bases, facial oedema, hepatomegaly, and less often splenomegaly or lymph node enlargement, were relatively common clinical signs during the first four weeks of the acute phase. Absolute eosinophilia (over 500 cells/ml) in peripheral blood was the most characteristic and reliable laboratory diagnostic index during this phase. In 15–18% of patients, the initial acute syndrome did not resolve.

Thus, in late June to early July 1981, some initial symptoms (constitutional symptoms, acute respiratory complaints, skin rashes) subsided, only to be replaced in the transitional period by new features, such as severe, diffuse myalgias, oedematous changes of the skin, dryness of the ocular and oral mucosae, progressive weight loss and, in some patients, thromboembolic complications.

Chronic phase: general features

The syndromes of the transitional period actually heralded the chronic phase of TOS, which was well defined from August 1981 onwards. This phase was characterized by an unprecedented combination of multisystemic symptoms and signs: peripheral neuropathy (mononeuropathy multiplex) with secondary widespread muscle wasting and deformity of the limbs, scleroderma-like and xerostomia/xerophthalmia syndromes, pulmonary hypertension and liver dysfunction. Less common features included oesophageal hypomotility and Raynaud's phenomenon. Myoclonias were a more recent (1983) serious neurological finding. Eosinophilia continued to be a typical laboratory index for more than 14 months, although with decreasing severity after August 1981. Thrombocytopenia was a relatively serious but transient haematological finding during the early period (July–August 1981) of the chronic phase (*6*). The occurrence of autoantibodies was occasionally reported during this late stage of TOS.

Thus, it is obvious that TOS encompassed a wide clinical spectrum, initially distinguished as a peculiar respiratory distress syndrome with severe constitutional symptoms and hypereosinophilia, that later developed into several systemic syndromes overlapping with variable intensity and prevalence in a relatively minor subset of the initial (more than 20 000) patient population.

Clinical symptoms and signs: specific features

Constitutional

Villamor León et al. (*7*) found that initially, only a minor fraction of patients (1.4%) was free of symptoms, but a complete lack of signs was not so uncommon (18.1%). Obviously, this changed dramatically in the ensuing weeks. Thus, at six months, 27.7% of patients were asymptomatic and 60% showed no signs. Of the early constitutional symptoms (e.g. asthenia, anorexia, fever, headache, weight loss) all but weight loss appeared with similar prevalence during the early chronic phase. Over the next few weeks, however, the occurrence of weight loss increased. Actually, in most of the hospital patients, weight loss progressed to severe undernutrition by June 1982.

In 86 patients at the Ramón y Cajal Centre whose clinical presentation started between 1 May and 15 June, the clinical features were similar to those described by Villamor León et al. (*7*), but with a higher incidence (total of about 92% with asthenia, malaise and/or anorexia as early symptoms), a greater general morbidity and an earlier and more severe weight loss (73%). On the other hand, weight loss in this population (64 out of 86 patients) was still mild (1–10 kg) in 50 cases, severe (10–15 kg) in only 10 cases, and exceptional (above 15 kg) in 4 patients. These results are at variance with the observations of some other groups that have reported a greater proportion of severe weight loss. A complete recovery of the pre-illness nutritional status after five months occurred in a significant proportion (36%) of the 86 patients, and a persistent or progressive course towards undernutrition was a rare event (8 cases, 9.3%). As could be expected under these circumstances, amenorrhoea was not uncommon (22%) but lasted no more than five months.

Cardiopulmonary

Along with the constitutional complaints described above, respiratory symptoms and signs dominated the clinical scene during the acute phase. Their prevalence during the first two months has been accurately reported by the Clinical Commission, including the data applied in retrospect to 1580 patients diagnosed from May to July 1981 (*8,9*). Haemoptysis is reported to have occurred in 7% of the patients of one hospital group (*5*). Most of the symptoms and signs of the acute phase disappeared after four months in 75–80% of patients. Dyspnoea as a result of mild activity still persisted in about 20% of patients after this time. On the other hand, abnormal auscultatory findings, either of the lung or the heart, were absent in more than 90% of patients by the fourth month. The chest X-ray changes have been well described by the Clinical Commission (*8,9*) and individual X-ray patterns by Cepeda et al. (*10*), who studied 884 patients diagnosed in the period from 5 May to 20 July 1981. According to these authors, there were three initial X-ray changes: interstitial, characterized by Kerley A and B lines, peribronchial oedema and posterior tracheal oedema; alveolar, with variable distribution as lobar (single/multiple), acinonodular, patchy (multiple), or butterfly-like; and pleural effusions that were either bilateral or unilateral of different localizations (e.g. fissures, subpulmonary) affecting one or both sides. A combination of these basic changes was often present. These changes were essentially the same as those reported by other groups, although the prevalence of individual X-ray patterns varied slightly from one to another. The interstitial radiological changes (Fig. 1), however, were found consistently by all groups to be the most common finding, followed by the pleural effusions. The alveolar changes were the least prevalent radiological pattern in most of the studies. All the changes were, as a whole, consistent with a noncardiogenic pulmonary oedema. The cardiothoracic index was normal in all reports. As happened with the clinical symptoms, the radiological changes that were present initially in virtually every patient were rather fleeting. Thus, about 87% of the patients had a normal X-ray by the 32nd week of TOS. This favourable evolution was spontaneous in some patients, but the role of the early steroid therapy had a significant influence in most of them (*10,11*).

Functional disturbances during the acute phase were several: moderate decrease in vital capacity in 26% of patients and in the forced expiratory volume in the first second (FEV_1) in 52% of the patients; abnormal diffusion tests (66%) and alteration in flux/volume curves (59.8%); and hypocapnia ascribed to both chronic hyperventilation and to a rise in the alveolar–arterial pO_2 gradient as reported by one group. Most of these alterations have slowly returned towards normality with the alveolar–arterial gradient parameter being the first to recover. In addition, the CO diffusion test has proved to be the most valuable method for following the evolution of the functional disturbance of the lung which, while having normalized in most of the affected patients by the end of 1982, still persists in about 10%. The most important haemodynamic impact of TOS has been pulmonary hypertension which started early in June 1981, affecting about 10% of the 1300 patients studied at that time (*8,9*).

Prominence of the pulmonary arterial cone in the chest X-ray (Fig. 2), ECG changes suggesting overload of the right ventricle and/or abnormal findings at physical examination of the heart (e.g. palpitation of the right ventricle, enhanced second heart tone) were the most prevalent signs pointing to pulmonary hypertension. Echographic and haemodynamic studies usually revealed a mild to moderate hypertension in most of the patients studied. In most of these cases, the pulmonary hypertension was not modified by oxygen or by drugs (e.g. calcium antagonists, steroids, platelet aggregation inhibitors, vasodilators) either alone or in different combinations. With time, pulmonary hypertension proved to be reversible in virtually all patients. Thus, the incidence of the disorder was found to be only 3.5% of a sample of 200 patients followed up by Gomez Recio et al. (*12*) in the period November/December 1982. In some of these patients, the main haemodynamic finding, although of questionable significance, was an increase in telediastolic pressure in the right ventricle.

Other cardiocirculatory disturbances have been rare. Arterial thromboembolism (mesenteric, pulmonary) has already been mentioned. Myocardial ischaemia and pericardial effusion have been reported in a small number of patients.

Digestive

Nonspecific digestive/abdominal symptoms were present in some 25–30% of patients during the acute phase of TOS (*7–9*). Nausea and vomiting were the more common early complaints and characteristically resolved in a few

Fig. 1. Typical bilateral diffuse interstitial changes seen in chest X-rays taken during the acute phase of TOS.

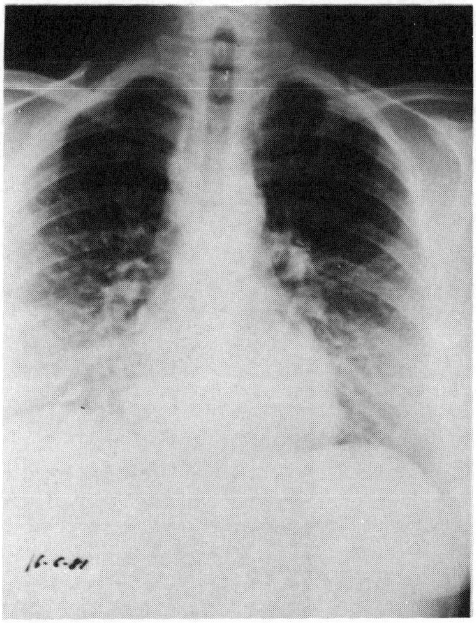

Fig. 2. Prominence of the pulmonary arterial cone with minimal residual bilateral lung changes due to pulmonary hypertension.

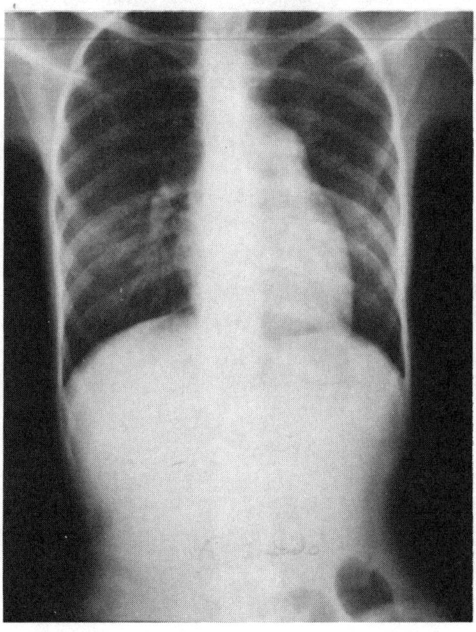

Fig. 3. Clawed hands in the chronic phase of TOS. The flexed fingers and atrophy of the interosseous muscle are typical.

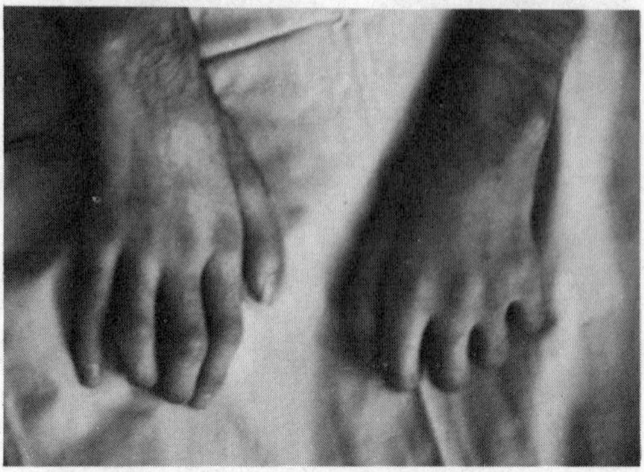

Fig. 4. Typical appearance of the flexed knee due to prolonged muscle atrophy and contracture in the chronic phase of TOS.

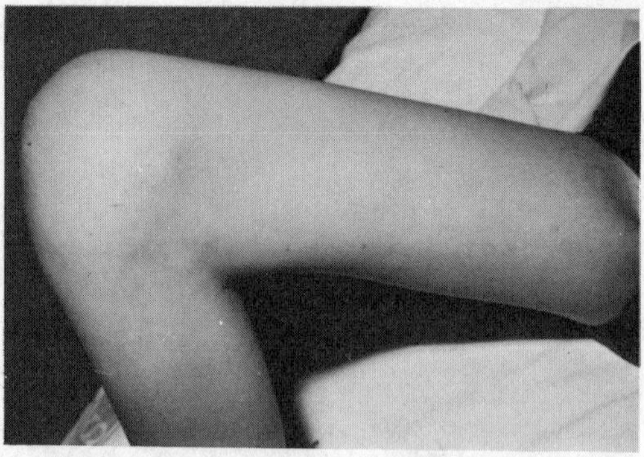

Fig. 5. Brittle, dystrophic nails with characteristic horizontal whitish streaks in the chronic phase of TOS.

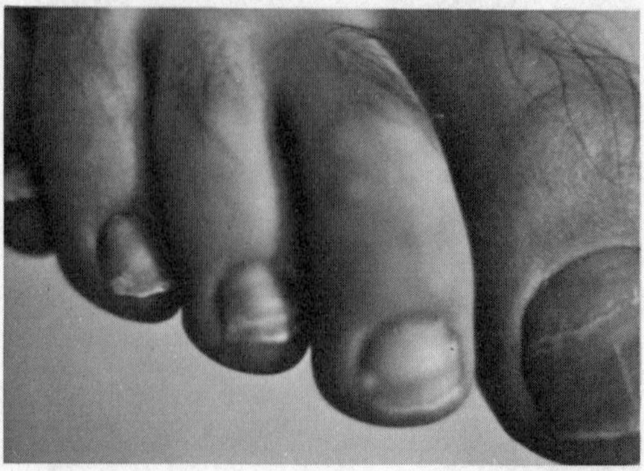

weeks. Dysphagia was initially described in 10–12% of patients, apparently due to abnormal peristalsis in the oesophagus. In the late phase, dysphagia (when present) was of multifactorial causation: dryness of the oral mucosa, neurogenic atrophy of the striated muscles of the oropharynx and/or fibrosis of the oesophageal wall. Abdominal pain was relatively common during the early phase, and in isolated cases clinical and biochemical evidence of pancreatitis was reported. Overt pancreatic pathology with exocrine/endocrine insufficiency was rare, however, despite the common fibrosis and atrophy of the gland found in most of the autopsied cases during the chronic phase of TOS. The reasons for this clinicopathological discrepancy are not known. The most interesting impact of TOS on the digestive system was the liver abnormalities, which affected an estimated 25–30% of the total population.

Interestingly, hepatomegaly was an early finding with normal liver biochemistry (transaminases, bilirubin, alkaline phosphatase) in nearly 100% of the patients. Later, two main biochemical patterns emerged in otherwise asymptomatic patients. One was an increase in transaminases (GOT/GPT), usually seen as a sequel to hepatic enlargement. The increase in transaminases was usually modest (less than four times the upper normal limit) and transient. Most of the cases were anicteric (82–84% in most of the series), and thus hyperbilirubinaemia was usually mild, slow to appear, and uncommon. The other pattern was cholestasis with or without hyperbilirubinaemia but typically expressed by increased serum levels of alkaline phosphatase and gamma-glutamyl transpeptidase. Lactate dehydrogenase was reported to be high in 84% of the patients in one study. Budd-Chiari syndrome has been described occasionally. The natural history of the cholestasis (*13, 14*) was more biochemical than clinical, with minor histological changes (see Pathology findings, p. 64) since the early phase and negligible progression in most of the cases that were rebiopsied after several months of development. A progression to histologically proven biliary cirrhosis has recently been reported. Interestingly, some workers have pointed out the virtual lack of previous alcoholic habits in most of these patients (*14*).

Neuromuscular

Retrospective studies (*15, 16*) have established neuromuscular damage as the most common (80%) and incapacitating clinical manifestation of TOS. The disease involved both the central and peripheral nervous systems with muscle damage mostly secondary to neuropathy, but the central nervous system has been relatively well preserved in most patients. According to one study at the Ramón y Cajal Centre (D. Muñoz et al., unpublished data) 12 out of 100 patients showed symptoms of encephalitis (impairment of consciousness, focal and generalized seizures) at the very onset of TOS and 48% showed spinal cord symptoms (myoclonias, fibrillations), pyramidal signs and/or changes in sensory level within the first three weeks of diagnosis of TOS.

These data are similar to those of the nationwide study by Portera (*17*) revealing diffuse encephalopathy with or without focal symptoms in 3–7%

of his patients. Portera also showed clinical features of cerebral ischaemia in 2–3% of the population, with only an occasional indication of an intracraneal high-pressure syndrome. All these alterations occurred early in the natural history of TOS (May–August 1981). More recently (June 1982), some suspected cases of Alzheimer-type encephalopathy have been claimed by some groups, but without convincing documentation. In contrast, peripheral nervous system damage was dominant in most patients (80% of all affected) according to Portera's estimates in June 1982, with a female : male ratio of 2 : 1 and with variable degrees of severity and persistence.

Two points deserve particular emphasis. First, intense and frequent (32.2%) myalgias still persisted in an important proportion of patients (34.4%) after six months. In other studies carried out at the Ramón y Cajal Centre (Muñoz et al. and Arechaga et al., unpublished data) myalgias were present in 60–64% of the patients within the first three weeks and in up to 80% in the first 13 weeks of the disease. They were usually widespread, with some preference for the paraspinal muscles and with increased severity during muscle palpation. Muscle cramps were initially uncommon but gradually appeared from the third to fourth week onwards, most often affecting the distal muscle groups. Loss of strength and muscle atrophy were readily apparent in the experience of all observers (*15,16*) from mid-July onwards and consistently progressed from August to October 1981, affecting 75% of the patients. A similar time course of changing patterns was established for muscle tone impairment, hyporeflexia and sensitivity alterations. Signs of autonomic neuropathy manifested by sinus tachycardia, reactive fixed mydriasis, postural hypotension and diffuse sweating disturbances (either hypo- or hyperhidrosis) were present in 87% of patients by the third week. In 47% of 100 patients (Muñoz et al., unpublished data) muscle wasting and generalized amyotrophy leading to permanent bed confinement and/or life-threatening respiratory failure was established from the seventh month to the time of writing (November 1981 — June 1982). Although muscle atrophy tended to be generalized, a characteristic distal pattern in the upper extremities (forearms and hands) with selective wasting of the interosseus muscle groups in the hands was most commonly observed in this stage (Fig. 3). Also in this stage, contractures were concomitant with muscle atrophy, affecting every region. Fixed flexed knees (Fig. 4), elbows or wrists and/or limited motion of the temporomandibular joints added further functional restriction, eventually leading to interference with vital activities, such as chewing and swallowing. Sensory alteration, though not so common, also increased over the months, particularly in those patients presenting the most severe atrophy. Electromyogram (EMG) changes were initially (in weeks 1–4) characterized by spontaneous fibrillations (91%) but with a mean duration of potentials within normal limits (82%), although a considerable proportion (60%) of patients exhibited polyphasic potentials. Gradually, EMG changes evolved into a pattern that consisted of increased spontaneous activity, decreased amplitude of the muscle potentials, and decreased conduction velocity in both the sensory and motor nerves in almost all patients.

This pattern heralded the progression towards generalized muscle wasting and severe contractures. In a one-year follow-up study of 100 patients (*16*), severe muscular involvement was still present in 15% of them, whereas a major proportion had minor (48%) to moderate (33%) involvement. Complete clinical remission was documented in only four patients. In the most advanced cases (in late 1982 and early 1983) abnormal movements added a further load to these severely handicapped patients: fasciculations, multifocal asymmetrical myoclonus, repetitive jerking, persistent muscle spasms (e.g. tongue, masseter muscle), tremors, or a complex combination of these abnormalities (*18*).

Mucocutaneous

The skin lesions in TOS typically changed from the acute to the chronic phase (*19*). About 70% of patients suffered cutaneous alterations during the early phase, either as irritative symptoms (pruritus, urticaria) or as polymorphic rashes (e.g. morbilliform or maculopapular exanthema). In addition, facial erythema and/or angioedema were common (30–60%). True purpura was rare. Most of these lesions were fleeting and self-limiting, disappearing in a few days. By the end of June 1981, 28–30% of patients developed nonpruriginous papular lesions overlapping with pasty oedema in several regions (face, abdomen, limbs) with or without diffuse brown pigmentation. In most patients, these changes progressed to unequivocal skin infiltration, leading in the following few months (September–December 1981) to the typical chronic phase consisting of scleroderma-like changes. In March 1982, about 80% of hospital patients had either localized or generalized sclerodermatous changes. A striking characteristic was that these skin changes were accompanied by severe neuromuscular disease in more than 80% of the patients and rarely (2% or less) appeared as an isolated alteration. In this late phase, skin changes were usually (75% or more of cases) concomitant with severe salivary and lacrimal hyposecretion (sicca syndrome) (*19,20*). Coincidence with other pathologies (pulmonary hypertension, liver disease) was less remarkable. Alopecia and nail dystrophy (Fig. 5) ran a comparable course. Other pathologies (of the lymphatic system, or the joints) occurred only occasionally. Arthralgias (*7*) were relatively common during the early phase (12%) and still persisted after a year in some patients.

In the chronic phase, joint deformities were common and usually secondary to several factors (neuromuscular and sclerodermatous pathological changes, prolonged immobilization, malnutrition). Contractures were common. In addition, radiological changes indicated severe diffuse osteoporosis in many patients.

Psychiatric

As the risk to health had such a brutal impact on the patients and the Spanish population in general, TOS could have been expected to elicit dramatic psychological reactions. In a thorough study conducted for the Clinical Commission (*21,22*) on 600 patients, however, anxiety and mild psychoaffective disorders, but no organic dementias, were found in about 90% of that population. Interestingly, antecedent psychiatric disorders were present in 55% of these patients, and in 32% of their families. Pregnancy did not appear to have a deleterious influence, and the reactive pattern in children was as could be expected for their ages.

Pregnancy
The influence of TOS on pregnancy has been carefully surveyed (*23,24*). No evidence of increased abortions, malformations or any other deleterious effects on the course and outcome of pregnancy has been detected in 300 women who had completed their pregnancy and delivered by June 1982.

Laboratory findings
Many biochemical abnormalities have been reported at the different stages of TOS. For an exhaustive discussion, we refer to some reliable sources (*5,25,26*). Only the most relevant data will be briefly mentioned here. Eosinophilia was the most specific marker of the syndrome, starting early (in the first week), progressively declining, and being present in 10% or less of the patients by March 1982. The biochemistry of the liver damage is also of interest and has been described earlier in this paper (p. 59).

An initial moderate leukocytosis (12 000/mm^3) appeared in 28% of cases in the first week (*25*) and was still observed in 11% of patients at the end of the fourth month. Lymphocytopenia and thrombocytopenia were marginal findings (22% of patients) during the first week, virtually disappearing after five months. No clotting disorders have been described as specifically due to TOS. Other biochemical findings included transient hypocholesterolaemia (15.4%) early in the onset of the disease and mild hypertriglycerinaemia. Hypoproteinaemia and hypoalbuminaemia (18.7% in the first week) returned to normal levels in most patients (48% of patients after six months). Rises in serum lactate dehydrogenase, initially present in 66.7% of patients, declined rapidly, and high levels of creatine phosphokinase and aldolase have occasionally been reported (*25,26*). A vast array of other enzymes has been assayed by various groups at different stages of TOS, but the results are only of marginal interest. Other biochemical and/or serological findings (hepatitis antigen, carcinoembryonic antigen, serum electrophoresis) were unremarkable. As a matter of fact, one is struck by the relative scarcity of enzymatic changes in such a devastating chronic disease, but this relative scarcity of enzymatic changes is consistent with the nature of a primary neuropathy with secondary muscle damage.

Immunology
The most clearcut finding during the acute phase was the common and significant elevation of IgE serum levels in many patients. Other immunological alterations were reported in small groups of patients by several groups during the acute phase, but their significance is doubtful. These include antibodies against many unrelated antigens (lung, T-lymphocytes) as well as modifications in the relative proportions of T-lymphocyte subpopulations (a decrease in T-suppressor cells). Most of these changes were fleeting and not reproducible in all the laboratories. During the late phase of TOS, most patients did not show any significant immunological alteration.

Antinuclear antibodies were detected in individual cases (4 out of 57 cases in studies at the Ramón y Cajal Centre) at low titres (1/80 and 1/320). Exceptionally, two cases were observed with significantly high titres (1/1280 and 1/10 240). Anti-smooth and -striated muscle antibodies and/or the presence of cryoglobulins or rheumatoid factor were only occasional findings. Among the most advanced cases (in late 1982 and early 1983) circulating immunocomplexes were detected only in some patients. No clinical or pathological correlations with any of the reported immunological findings could be established (*27,28*). A single study on human lymphocyte antigen phenotyping in patients during the chronic phase reported an increase of DR3/DR4 frequencies in the most affected female patients (*29,30*). Further confirmation of this finding is needed. Other studies reporting the possible presence of anti-oleilanilide activity in the sera of severe chronic cases are interesting, but this possibility requires further confirmation.

In summary, except for the early transient elevation in serum IgE levels, immunological changes throughout the natural history of TOS were scant, bizarre and hard to interpret.

Clinical management and treatment

This aspect has been one of the most frustrating of this new disease. Owing to the overwhelming number of new cases and the total ignorance about the cause and physiopathology of the disorders, physicians were initially both surprised and disoriented. According to the rapidly changing interpretations of the pathogenesis of the syndrome (infection with bacteria or mycoplasmata; allergic disorder) a battery of remedies, usually different from hospital to hospital, was used. Because the infection hypothesis was held by many, the antibiotic erythromycin was used on many patients for a short period of 2–3 weeks at the beginning of the epidemic. As soon as a hypersensitivity reaction was suggested in early May by the striking eosinophilia, steroids (mostly methylprednisolone and prednisone) were used, either alone or in combination with the antibiotic or with other drugs. Agreement is unanimous that the use of steroids during that early phase was particularly efficacious in improving the clinical and radiological symptoms of respiratory involvement (*10,11*). As shown by some groups, the clinical and radiological response to steroids was virtually immediate and spectacular in most cases. The influence of the early steroid treatment on the long-term outcome of the syndrome has been difficult to establish, but according to some groups, a good prognosis followed an early complete response to the drug (*4–6,31*).

A significant proportion (15–18%) of patients, however, entered the chronic phase despite various dosages and schedules of steroid administration. In addition, it is beyond doubt that once the patient entered the chronic phase, particularly if neuromuscular and dermal changes were severe, the efficacy of steroids diminished and they were eventually contraindicated in the most advanced cases. Therefore, from late 1982 to early 1983, these compounds were used only in very special circumstances. Other drug regimens were introduced, not only when the association of the syndrome with the ingestion of toxic oils was proved, but as each new pathogenetic hypothesis emerged (e.g. autoimmunity, free radical generation). Immunosuppressor drugs (azathioprine), radical scavengers (superoxide dismutase, tryptophan, dimethyl sulfoxide), vitamin E, D-penicillamine, L-carnitine and some other drugs (*16,32*) were therefore used by many different groups, usually on a limited number of patients during the chronic phase.

A critical analysis of these therapeutic attempts, which have been summarized elsewhere, is beyond the aims of this paper. To say that all these measures have only marginal, if any, importance may very well summarize our view. Further, other "therapies" have sometimes been anecdotal. Plasmapheresis has been tried in a few cases (in the chronic phase) without success. On the other hand, after the initial relief provided by the steroids during the acute phase, many disabled patients during the chronic phase of TOS greatly benefited from well conducted physiotherapy programmes (*33*), psychological support and several symptomatic measures, such as sedatives, tranquillizers and relaxant drugs.

Pathology findings

Our present knowledge of the pathological changes associated with TOS is reasonably complete and accurate despite the relatively scarce number of biopsy and/or autopsy studies so far performed (*34–36*). Most of the description presented here is based on the reports of the National Programme for the Toxic Syndrome and on the comprehensive published works of Martinez Tello et al. (*36*).

General histopathological features

Three basic lesional patterns underlay the complex clinical spectrum of TOS: vascular damage; interstitial inflammatory infiltrates and/or fibrosis; and atrophy of affected organs. Fibrosis and organ (parenchyma) atrophy evolved slowly, were widespread, and increased in severity as the late chronic phase of the syndrome progressed. On the other hand, vascular lesions were the hallmark of TOS throughout the entire natural history of the syndrome. This particular aspect of the histopathology of the syndrome is therefore described here in some detail.

Lesional patterns of vascular damage. Virtually any vessel regardless of its size and/or anatomical structure in almost any tissue could be affected at any time. Despite the ubiquity of the vascular damage, TOS showed a predilection for vascular beds in the lungs, skin, skeletal muscle and peripheral nerves. The central nervous system and the kidneys were often spared, even in severely affected patients.

Two categories of elementary lesion contributed to the vascular pathology of TOS: degenerative (cellular swelling, cytoplasmic vacuolization, necrosis of endothelial cells) and proliferative changes in the vascular endothelium. Often these changes combined with different degrees of "aggressiveness" and led to occlusion (partial or total) of the lumen of the vessels (Fig. 6).

Non-necrotizing, nongranulomatous vasculitis. The infiltrates were either perivascular or confined to the media and/or the intima layers of the vessel

Fig. 6. Proliferative changes at the intima leading to virtual occlusion of the lumen of a pulmonary arteriole.

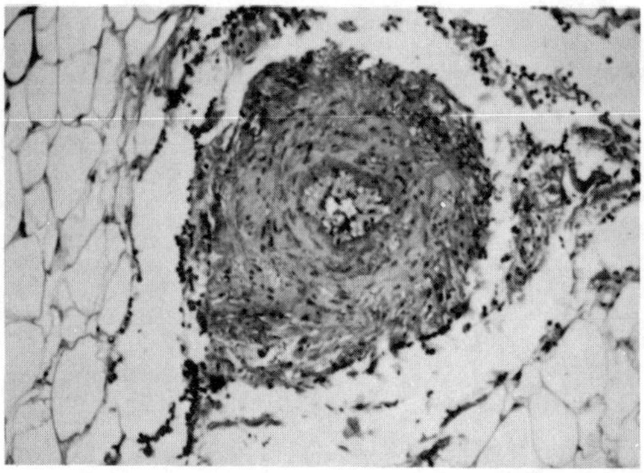

Fig. 7. Fibrosis and detachment of the intima in a pulmonary arteriole. The elastic layer is intact.

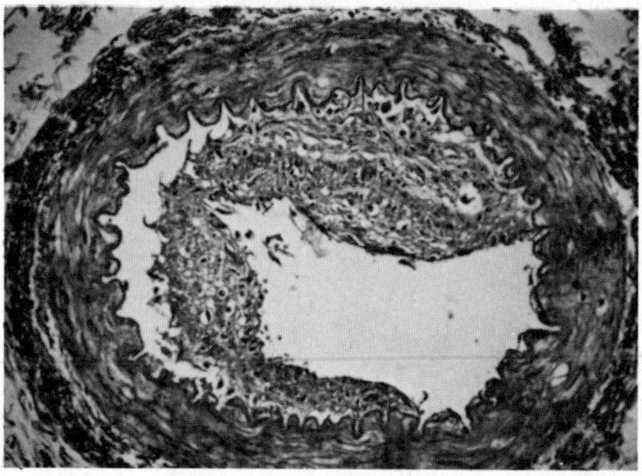

Fig. 8. Parietal changes in an arteriole. Note the "foamy cells" and slight perivascular infiltration.

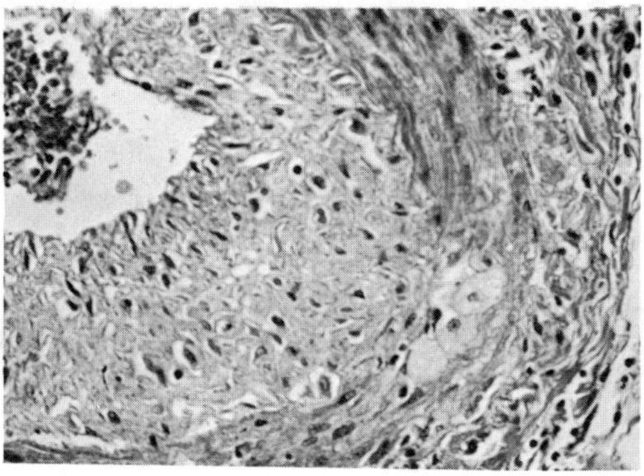

Fig. 9. Perineural fibrosis in a peripheral nerve in the chronic phase of TOS. Note the random damage to nerve bundles.

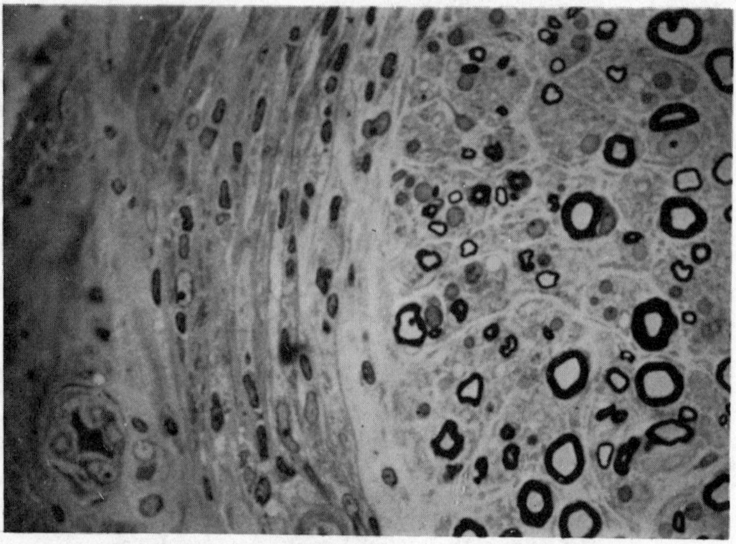

Fig. 10. Muscle biopsy (reverse ATPase stain) showing changes compatible with type II fibre atrophy.

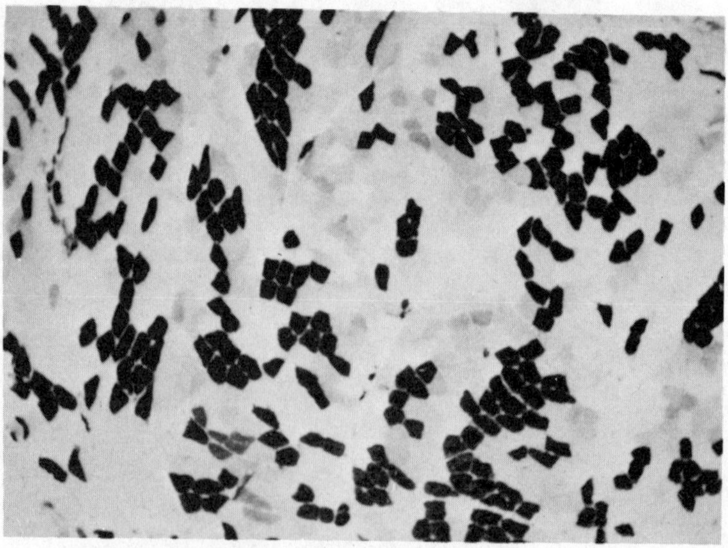

wall. The perivascular infiltrates were found almost exclusively during the acute clinical phase of TOS, gradually fading until they virtually disappeared in the chronic phase of the syndrome. Infiltration of the media was less common but could be detected at any step in the natural history of the syndrome. The most typical pattern was, indeed, that of endarteritis and/or endophlebitis with the inflammatory changes tending to be more severe in the subendothelial space. In each of these patterns, the infiltrates comprised mixed cells: lymphocytes, histiocytes and eosinophils. Less often, polymorphonuclear leukocytes were also present.

Intimal fibrosis and vessel occlusion. These lesions occurred mainly in the chronic phase of TOS and were probably the final common pathway of endothelial damage, wall infiltration and excessive proliferative activity of fibroblasts and/or myofibroblasts at the intima. Irregular narrowing of the vessel lumen and partial or total intimal detachment were common concomitant features (Fig. 7). In much advanced lesions, vacuolated cells (histiocytes?) with a peculiar "foamy" appearance were often found within the frame of the proliferated intima. The significance and nature of these cells are unknown (Fig. 8).

Thromboembolic complications. These have been reported to happen at any stage of TOS. Typically occurring in the lung during the acute phase, other vascular beds (mesenteric/portal veins and mesenteric/femoral/carotid arteries) were the preferred sites as the syndrome progressed into the transitional and chronic clinical phases.

Special pathology

The lungs. These organs were the typical target at the earliest stages of TOS, and this was mistakenly interpreted on clinical and radiological grounds as "atypical pneumonia". At those stages, autopsy findings were the following: diffuse septal oedema and light to mild interstitial mixed cell (mononuclear cells, scattered eosinophils) infiltration; discrete changes in pneumonocytes (cuboidal metaplasia of type II cells, diminished proportion and alveolar desquamation of type I cells) and alveolar desquamation (macrophages, type I cells) with oedema; and vascular changes as described earlier and, occasionally, lymphangiectasia in the interlobular septa.

In the chronic phase of the syndrome, vasculitis in the lung (as in other organs) dominated the pathological spectrum. Many autopsies showed, however, that mild (less often severe) inflammatory changes persisted even in the most advanced cases. Interestingly, fibrosis was not a pathological finding in the lung even in those patients who showed severe dysfunction with or without pulmonary hypertension.

Peripheral nerves, central nervous system and skeletal muscle. The evolving spectrum of the peripheral nerve damage has been well characterized (*36,37*) through the systematic study of tissue samples from biopsies and/or autopsies mostly performed during the transitional and chronic phases of the syndrome. According to Tellez et al. (*37*) early lesions consisted of severe perineuritis (mixed-cell perivascular infiltrates) with a severity that varied from one nerve fascicle to another and a peculiar predilection for distal over proximal nerves. At any rate, the most consistent findings were of epi- and perineural lymphocytic infiltration and loss of the thick myelinated fibres with marked disruption of the remaining myelin sheaths (splitting, vacuolization, distension). Later, these alterations were slowly replaced by severe perineural fibrosis of focal distribution. Martinez Tello et al. (*36*) reported this later finding in 43% of the biopsies examined and in all the autopsies performed during the chronic phase of the syndrome. Total nerve fibre degeneration (axonal loss, myelin clumping, collapsed axons, wallerian degeneration) unequally affecting the different nerve fascicles (Fig. 9) was a rather constant feature of the late phase. Remarkably, the Schwann cells remained intact or were only minimally damaged. The unmyelinated nerve fibres were usually spared. Although a good clinicopathological correlation was found in most of the studies, some patients had severe pathological changes in the peripheral nerves, with minimal or no clinical or neurological symptoms.

In contrast to the peculiar vulnerability of the peripheral nerves, the central nervous system seemed to be relatively resistant to the impact of TOS. Most of the reported lesions were, indeed, late in appearing, nonspecific in character, and most probably had a multifactorial cause (ischaemic, nutritional and other factors) rather than being linked to the presumed offending agent(s) in TOS. Perivascular round cell infiltrates in the leptomeninges and/or in the parenchyma along with ischaemic lesions (microinfarcts) were reported in relatively early cases (in July/August 1981). Most often, these lesions were found in patients dying in the advanced stages of the disease. Chromatolysis of the motor neurons in the spinal cord and the pons, as well as in the substantia reticularis of the medulla and the nuclei of cranial nerves V and VII, has also been reported.

The skeletal muscle was involved from the earliest stages of TOS. According to Tellez et al. (*37*), the initial muscle damage was an inflammatory myopathy. Mild to moderate mixed cell (lymphocytes, histiocytes, eosinophils) perifascicular and perimysial inflammation with no fibre necrosis was seen early in the syndrome and in the transitional (myalgia) period. Endomysial inflammation was uncommon, tending to be localized around the muscle, spindle and the intramuscular nerve fibres. Histochemistry (Fig. 10) has shown that changes (reverse ATPase stain) compatible with predominant or exclusive type II fibre atrophy can be detected at a relatively early stage. As the syndrome progressed and muscle wasting increased in severity, a typical histopathological muscle pattern emerged. This consisted of widespread denervation, atrophy, and marked endoperimysial fibrosis in the most severely affected patients. Virtually every muscle, including the diaphragm and intercostal groups, was found to be damaged in most of the autopsied cases who died during the chronic phase. A predominantly proximal over distal muscle pattern distribution was maintained even at this stage. Whereas the secondary myopathy of the chronic phase is a rather nonspecific picture, the early myopathy in TOS (*37*) may be distinguished from that found in connective tissue diseases (e.g. lupus erythematosus) or in polymyositis by the lack of myofibril necrosis, fibre regeneration and endomysial damage.

Mucocutaneous system. The main features in the acute and chronic phases were clearly different even though some alterations have been reported that are common to both. The histopathological changes detected during the acute phase of TOS were confined to the dermis, while the epidermis remained untouched or had only minor abnormalities, such as focal spongiosis or exocytosis. Changes to the dermis were of four types.

1. *Perivascular lymphohistiocytic infiltrates* of varying degrees of severity occurred mainly at the superficial dermal plexus. Occasionally, similar findings were observed around the deeper dermal plexus. Eosinophils and sometimes neutrophils, plasma and mast cells were also found.

2. Also present were *changes of the vascular endothelium* (tumefaction, swelling, mitotic figures) and dilated lumina with foci of agglutinated erythrocytes. More often these changes coexisted with scattered clumps of extravasated red cells.

3. *Oedema* (slight to moderate) of dermal papillae tended to fade away with no sequelae in a significant proportion of patients. In those who entered the systemic chronic phase of TOS, however, the spectrum of the skin changes evolved into a more peculiar histopathological picture. Interstitial inflammatory infiltration (essentially perpetuating those alterations seen in the early acute phase) in some particularly severe cases distorted the alignment and boundaries of the dermal collagen fibres. Gradually, the inflammatory changes were replaced by fibrosclerosis due to collagen fibre proliferation of variable intensity, leading to thickened collagen bundles that occupied the reticular dermis and eventually extended to the hypodermis.

4. Finally, *mucinosis* detected at the beginning of the chronic phase (August 1981) was superimposed on the fibrosclerotic changes. Vasculitis was very common (61% of biopsies in Martinez Tello's study (*36*)) in the chronic phase with characteristics identical to those found elsewhere.

In addition to these four elementary lesions, others of lesser incidence were added. Tissue eosinophilia, according to Martinez Tello (*36*), was present in 33% of the biopsies during the chronic phase as compared with 73% in the skin samples examined during the acute phase. Also present were fusiform cells that were identified by light microscopy and most clearly by their ultrastructural pictures (showing electron-dense fibril-like inclusion bodies) as probably corresponding to activated fibroblasts. Finally, distortion of elastic fibres and perineural infiltrations were found, similar to those seen around the nerves in other localizations.

Liver and bile system. As already described, liver disease in TOS was more biochemical than clinical, but it is still one of the most common and interesting aspects of the systemic pathology of this syndrome. Although no satisfactory, well controlled prospective studies are yet available, it seems that the lesional pattern of the liver in TOS was wide, ranging from minimal damage to severe cholestasis (minor proportion). Its morphological characteristics, however, are essentially those described in toxic hepatitis (*14*) due to various offending agents. The most detailed description comes from biopsies obtained during the early (May–July 1981) and transitional (July 1981) phases of TOS (*13,14*).

Early changes in the liver have been well described by Solís Herruzo et al. (*13*) who studied the liver biopsies of 24 patients diagnosed with TOS in May and June 1981, after 10–20 days of suspected exposure to toxic oil. Two types of lesion were found: portal and lobular. Mixed cell (histiocytes, polymorphonuclear lymphocytes, eosinophils) infiltration of the portal area, along with the spotty acidophilic degeneration of hepatocytes, was the most common picture. Other lesions included damage to the epithelium of the bile duct (11 out of 24 cases), portal venulitis (9 out of 24 cases) and marginal changes (4 out of 24 cases) which included swelling of the hepatic artery endothelium, enhanced reticulin framework and cholestasis. Several ultrastructural features added to this complex picture: giant mitochondria with parachrystalline inclusions, hyperplasia of the smooth endoplasmic reticulum, lamellar bodies in hepatocytes and Kupffer cells, and diverse lesions of the biliary pole of hepatocytes. Progression of the liver changes seemed to be slow or tended to stabilize. Although sequential studies are scarce, it seems that progression to liver cirrhosis has not been convincingly shown or is exceptional if it ever occurs.

More recently, isolated cases of rebiopsied patients have presented histological evidence of either "piecemeal necrosis" with variable degrees of fibrosis, or changes compatible with biliary cirrhosis after prolonged clinical/biological cholestasis. Evidence of immunopathological damage is lacking.

Kidneys. Clinically, renal involvement in TOS was rather uncommon, and significant pathological changes were exceptional. Only Gutierrez Millet et al. (*38*) have reported four cases of TOS apparently with no previous renal disease, who showed severe kidney damage at autopsy. The histological and immunopathological kidney lesions in these patients corresponded to diffuse endocapillary, membranoproliferative, and diffuse extracapillary glomerulonephritis. Most of the studies, however, have reported either no changes or only mild interstitial inflammatory changes and vasculitis.

Other organs. Since the impact of TOS eventually reached every system, other organ lesions may also have been present. In the heart, typical features of nonbacterial thrombotic endocarditis, mostly of the right side, have been described in both the early and late clinical phases. Myocarditis may be concomitant with it or appear as an independent finding. Severe stenosis of a coronary artery due to typical vasculitis changes was reported in a 12-year-old girl dying from chronic TOS. Fibrotic changes and marked atrophy of the pancreas, salivary glands and thyroid were common during the late phase.

Conclusions

1. The pathological hallmarks of the syndrome were of peculiar ubiquity and lesional pattern and comprised endothelial degeneration/proliferation, non-necrotizing nongranulomatous vasculitis, and a tendency to occlusion and/or thromboembolization of blood vessels.

2. The tendency was towards interstitial inflammatory infiltration in most organs, coupled with progressive severe fibrosis eventually contributing to organ atrophy. This behaviour was particularly characteristic of the skin, the peripheral nerves and certain internal organs (pancreas, salivary glands, thyroid).

3. The target organs varied with time, but eventually the impact of TOS became systemic. The lung was the major target organ during the first clinical phase (1 May — 15 June 1981) suffering a combination of lesions better described as noncardiogenic inflammatory oedema. Thromboembolism was common in this phase. Later, during the second (July–December 1981) and sequelae phases (January 1982 to the present) the neuromuscular system and the skin were the most severely affected target systems. A complex histopathological syndrome, compatible with multiple mononeuropathy, caused by perineural fibrosis and nerve fibre loss, with secondary muscle atrophy, illustrated the neurological damage. Vascular damage (non-necrotizing vasculitis) of small arteries in the hypodermis and dermo-epidermo-fibrosclerosis were the essential histopathological components of the late scleroderma-like syndrome of TOS.

In summary, TOS has had a major impact on health in Spain with entirely unique clinical and pathological characteristics. Its peculiar natural history means that TOS is, indeed, a new disease or syndrome of diseases. By contrast with the fairly complete knowledge of the clinicopathological aspects of TOS available at present, its precise cause and pathogenesis still remain a mystery.

References

1. **Tabuenca, J.M.** Toxic-allergic syndrome caused by ingestion of rapeseed oil denatured with aniline. *Lancet,* **2**: 567–568 (1981).
2. **Rigau-Perez, J.G. et al.** Estudios epidemiológicos sobre el síndrome tóxico en Navas del Marques (Avila) [Epidemiological studies on the toxic syndrome in Navas del Marques (Avila)]. *In: Simposium Nacional "Síndrome Tóxico" [National Symposium on the Toxic Syndrome], Madrid, 11–12 June 1982.* Madrid, Ministry of Health and Consumer Affairs, 1982, pp. 217–219.

3. **Catalá Villanueva, F.J. & Mata de la Torre, J.M.S.** Epidemiología del síndrome tóxico [Epidemiology of the toxic syndrome]. *In: Simposium Nacional "Síndrome Tóxico" [National Symposium on the Toxic Syndrome], Madrid, 11–12 June 1982.* Madrid, Ministry of Health and Consumer Affairs, 1982, pp. 143–149.
4. **Tabuenca, J.M. et al.** Algunos aspectos del estado actual de los conocimientos del síndrome tóxico [Some aspects of the actual state of knowledge of the toxic syndrome]. *Nuevos archivos de la Facultad de Medicina,* **41**: 225–228 (1983).
5. **Toxic Epidemic Syndrome Study Group.** Toxic epidemic syndrome, Spain, 1981. *Lancet,* **2**: 697–702 (1982).
6. **Gilsanz, V.** Late features of the toxic syndrome due to denatured rapeseed oil. *Lancet,* **1**: 335–336 (1982).
7. **Villamor León, J. et al.** Descripción clínica de la enfermedad en adultos [Clinical description of the illness in adults]. *In: Simposium Nacional "Síndrome Tóxico" [National Symposium on the Toxic Syndrome], Madrid, 11–12 June 1982.* Madrid, Ministry of Health and Consumer Affairs, 1982, pp. 47–73.
8. **López Encuentra, A. et al.** Patología pulmonar [Pulmonary pathology]. *In: Simposium Nacional "Síndrome Tóxico" [National Symposium on the Toxic Syndrome], Madrid, 11–12 June 1982.* Madrid, Ministry of Health and Consumer Affairs, 1982, pp. 181–184.
9. *Cardiopulmonary pathology in the toxic syndrome.* Copenhagen, WHO Regional Office for Europe, 1983 (unpublished document ICP/RCE 905(1)/9).
10. **Cepeda, M.T. et al.** Hallazgos radiológicos pulmonares en la fase aguda del síndrome del aceite tóxico (S.A.T.) [Pulmonary radiological discoveries in the acute phase of the toxic oil syndrome]. *Nuevos archivos de la Facultad de Medicina,* **41**: 229–236 (1983).
11. **de la Cruz Rios, J. et al.** Estudio evolutivo de la radiología torácica en el síndrome tóxico. Análisis de la respuesta al tratamiento corticoide [Developmental studies of thoracic radiology in the toxic syndrome. Analysis of results of corticoid treatment]. *Revista clínica española,* **169**: 37–41 (1983).
12. **Gomez Recio, M. et al.** Hipertensión pulmonar en el síndrome tóxico [Pulmonary hypertension in the toxic syndrome]. *Nuevos archivos de la Facultad de Medicina,* **41**: 237–244 (1983).
13. **Solís Herruzo, J.A. et al.** Hepatopatía en el síndrome tóxico por consumo de aceite adulterado en el área de Madrid [Hepatology of the toxic syndrome due to consumption of adulterated oil in the area of Madrid]. *Gastroenterología y hepatología,* **5**: 113–124 (1982).
14. **Velicia, R. et al.** La hepatopatía del síndrome tóxico por aceite tóxico [The hepatology of the toxic syndrome due to toxic oil]. *Gastroenterología y hepatología,* **5**: 125–130 (1982).
15. **Ministry of Health and Consumer Affairs.** *Summary of activities of the Study Group for Neurological Manifestations of the Toxic Oil Syndrome.* Copenhagen, WHO Regional Office for Europe, 1983 (unpublished document ICP/RCE 905(1)/8).

16. **Portera Sánchez, A. et al.** Neuromuscular manifestations of the toxic oil syndrome in Spain. *In:* Battistin, L. et al., ed. *Clinical and biological aspects of the peripheral nervous system diseases.* New York, Alan R. Liss (in press).
17. **Portera Sánchez, A.** *Síndrome tóxico. Patología neurológica* [Toxic syndrome. Neurological pathology]. *In: Simposium Nacional "Síndrome Tóxico" [National Symposium on the Toxic Syndrome], Madrid, 11–12 June 1982.* Madrid, Ministry of Health and Consumer Affairs, 1982, pp. 127–131.
18. **Legg, N.J. & Marsden, C.D.** *Toxic oil syndrome. Report on a visit to Madrid, 26–28 October 1982.* Copenhagen, WHO Regional Office for Europe, 1983 (unpublished document ICP/RCE 903).
19. **Fonseca Capdevila, E. et al.** Manifestaciones cutáneas del síndrome tóxico por aceite adulterado [Cutaneous manifestations of the toxic syndrome due to adulterated oil]. *In: Simposium Nacional "Síndrome Tóxico" [National Symposium on the Toxic Syndrome], Madrid, 11–12 June 1982.* Madrid, Ministry of Health and Consumer Affairs, 1982, pp. 138–142.
20. *Dermatology.* Copenhagen, WHO Regional Office for Europe, 1983 (unpublished document ICP/RCE 905(1)/13).
21. **Sorio, J. et al.** Aspectos psiquiátricos del síndrome tóxico [Psychiatric aspects of the toxic syndrome]. *In: Simposium Nacional "Síndrome Tóxico" [National Symposium on the Toxic Syndrome], Madrid, 11–12 June 1982.* Madrid, Ministry of Health and Consumer Affairs, 1982, pp. 338–345.
22. *Psychiatry and the toxic syndrome.* Copenhagen, WHO Regional Office for Europe, 1983 (unpublished document ICP/RCE 905(1)/25).
23. **Nema, C. et al.** *Results of a prospective study of 32 newborns from mothers affected by the Spanish toxic syndrome (STS).* Copenhagen, WHO Regional Office for Europe, 1983 (unpublished document ICP/RCE 905(1)/19).
24. *Obstetric/gynecological pathology and the toxic syndrome due to adulterated colza oil.* Copenhagen, WHO Regional Office for Europe, 1983 (unpublished document ICP/RCE 905(1)/18).
25. *Biochemistry and the toxic syndrome.* Copenhagen, WHO Regional Office for Europe, 1983 (unpublished document ICP/RCE 905(1)/21).
26. **Coca, C. et al.** Screening de pacientes en el síndrome tóxico [Screening of patients with toxic syndrome]. *In: Simposium Nacional "Síndrome Tóxico" [National Symposium on the Toxic Syndrome], Madrid, 11–12 June 1982.* Madrid, Ministry of Health and Consumer Affairs, 1982, pp. 425–428.
27. *Summary of the immunological findings in the toxic syndrome.* Copenhagen, WHO Regional Office for Europe, 1983 (unpublished document ICP/RCE 905(1)/11).
28. **Bootello, A.** *Immunological studies on the toxic oil syndrome.* Copenhagen, WHO Regional Office for Europe, 1983 (unpublished document ICP/RCE 905(1)/12).

29. **Vicario, J.L. et al.** HLA-DR3,DR4 increase in chronic stage of Spanish oil disease. *Lancet,* **1**: 276 (1982).
30. **Vicario, J.L. et al.** *Chronic stage of the Spanish rapeseed oil disease. A new HLA-linked syndrome.* Madrid, Head Council of Scientific Investigations, 1983, Vol. 2.
31. **Barbadillo García Velasco, R. et al.** Tratamiento corticoideo de la afectación neuromuscular en la enfermedad tras ingesta de aceite de colza desnaturalizado [Corticoid treatment of the neuromuscular disorder in the illness resulting from ingestion of denatured colza oil]. *In: Simposium Nacional "Síndrome Tóxico" [National Symposium on the Toxic Syndrome], Madrid, 11–12 June 1982.* Madrid, Ministry of Health and Consumer Affairs, 1982, pp. 601–608.
32. *Therapeutic aspects of the toxic syndrome.* Copenhagen, WHO Regional Office for Europe, 1983 (unpublished document ICP/RCE 905(1)/26).
33. **Pastrana, R. et al.** Aspectos rehabilitadores del síndrome tóxico por aceite adulterado [Rehabilitation aspects of the toxic syndrome due to adulterated oil]. *In: Simposium Nacional "Síndrome Tóxico" [National Symposium on the Toxic Syndrome], Madrid, 11–12 June 1982.* Madrid, Ministry of Health and Consumer Affairs, 1982, pp. 635–640.
34. *Pathology of the toxic syndrome (TS) caused by ingestion of adulterated oil.* Copenhagen, WHO Regional Office for Europe, 1983 (unpublished document ICP/RCE 905(1)/17).
35. Report of the Pathology Commission of the Minister of Health. *Boletín epidemiológico semanal,* **1503**: 297–299 (1981).
36. **Martinez Tello, F.J. et al.** Pathology of a new toxic syndrome caused by ingestion of adulterated oil in Spain. *Virchows Archiv. A: pathological anatomy and histology,* **397**(3): 261–285 (1982).
37. **Tellez, I. et al.** *Neuropathology of the toxic syndrome caused by adulterated rapeseed oil,* Vol. 2. Madrid, Head Council of Scientific Investigations, 1983.
38. **Gutierrez Millet, V. et al.** Renal involvement in toxic syndrome. *Lancet,* **1**: 19–20 (1982).

Annex 4

Analysis and refining of aniline-denatured rapeseed oil

G.K.Koch

When in early autum 1981, personnel at Unilever Research Laboratorium in the Netherlands were asked by WHO to act as advisers, it was becoming a fairly general assumption that fatty acid anilides were indicative of toxic oils and indeed were the causal agents. Several internal meetings of scientific and technical experts were held at Unilever to consider the following questions: what refining procedures might have been applied to the aniline-denatured oil; at what stage(s) in the handling and processing of the oil might fatty acid anilides have been formed; and what other types of compound might be formed by reactions of aniline under the likely handling and processing conditions?

To tackle these questions, the author was invited by WHO to visit Spain as an adviser and Unilever decided to do a few processing/analytical experiments to check some of the ideas that had emerged. The conclusions they reached were sent to WHO.

In this paper, a summary is made of the results of analytical activities, carried out mainly in Spain but also in some other countries, to characterize suspect oils and to try to detect the components or contaminants that might have been responsible for the toxic oil syndrome. Then, there is a description of some possible reactions of aniline in, and with, an oil during storage and processing and the wide variety of possible products apart from the well known anilides. Finally, there is a discussion of the various procedures for oil processing or refining that may have been applied to the suspect oil and the results of some of the model experiments carried out by Unilever.

Analysis of oil composition and contamination

The characterization of the components of oil was made by the normal procedures of fatty acid analysis by gas-liquid chromatography (GLC) and sterol analysis of the unsaponifiable fraction of the oil by thin-layer chromatography (TLC) and/or GLC. For example, brassicasterol is used as an indicator for the presence of rapeseed oil and cholesterol for the presence of animal fat. The Institute of Fats and their Derivatives in Seville, especially, has been very active in the field of characterizing the composition of suspect samples of oil.

Most of the effort on contaminant analysis has been concentrated on the identification and determination of aniline and fatty acid anilides. Numerous oil samples have been analysed by the National Centre for Food and Nutrition in Majadahonda and the Institute of Fats and their Derivatives in Seville, using a GLC-finish for quantification. Methods have been developed in other countries, leading to reliable screening for low levels of anilide contamination (<1 ppm) (*1–3*).

Traces of other aromatic compounds that are probably related to the presence of aniline, such as azobenzene, methylaniline, bromoaniline, formanilide, quinoline, nitrobenzene and bromodiazobenzene have been detected in a number of oil samples. Other possibly dangerous contaminants, such as heavy metals, organochlorine and organophosphorus pesticides, mineral oils, artificial colourants, aflatoxins or polychlorinated biphenyls, have been sought but not detected. Apparently, microbiological contamination of any form can also be excluded. The presence of other compounds, such as the weedkiller paraquat, was suggested but later rejected. Recently, the presence of chloropropanediol esters (*4,5*) (and of reaction products of aniline and anilides such as iminoquinones and phenyl isocyanates) has been reported, but they do not seem to be obvious candidates for the observed toxic phenomena. In fact, up until now, no known chemical has been associated with the extraordinary character of the disease.

At the moment, it appears that all truly case-related oil samples consist largely of rapeseed oil mixed with some animal fat and grapeseed oil and contain traces of aniline and 1000–2000 ppm of fatty acid anilides.

Analytical limitations

Three factors have combined to limit the contribution of analytical chemistry to elucidating the cause of TOS. First, the poor system and procedures of identification and documentation of suspect oils during their collection and storage have led to great difficulty in establishing whether or not particular oil samples were actually case-related and, therefore, to much wasted effort and irrelevant data. Second, the failure to develop early enough a biological toxicity screening test conclusively correlated with the disease has made it impossible to validate whether particular oil samples or fractions from them are related to TOS. It has therefore been impossible to mount a systematic programme of analysis, isolation and identification. Indeed, Aldridge & Connors (*6*) have recently described the failure of a variety of animal and cell toxicity tests to show a response to the oils, at least some of which were believed to be case-related, which suggests that some unstable compound, no longer present in the oil, may have been the toxic agent. Third, the rather early identification of significant amounts of fatty acid anilides in many samples of suspect oils led to a fairly general assumption that these compounds were the toxic agents. This, in turn, led to too great a concentration of analytical (as well as biomedical) resources on the study of these compounds alone, at the expense of broader, more open-minded and probably more relevant studies.

Possible reactions of aniline in vegetable oil

From theoretical considerations as well as from experimental studies in Spain, it is clear that apart from fatty acid anilides, a wide variety of other products can be formed in an oil, especially in the presence of a considerable amount of linoleic acid-containing glycerides.

Experimental studies to date have concentrated almost exclusively on reaction products of aniline on its own and of fatty acid anilides. At the National Centre for Food and Nutrition in Majadahonda, mass spectrometry identified the compound 2,5-dianilino-*p*-benzoiminoquinone, which appeared to be highly toxic in a cell culture test and which may be hydrolysed to the benzoquinone derivative:

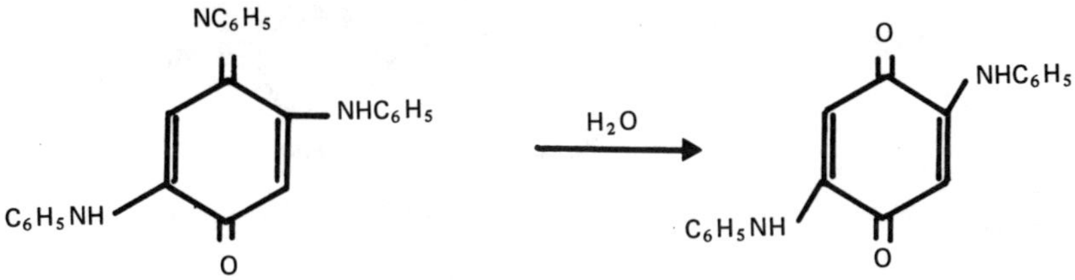

Acid anilides can be converted by heating into phenyl isocyanates ($C_6H_5N{=}C{=}O$), which were found to be toxic in a cell culture test at a level as low as 10 ppm (*5*). Pestaña & Muñoz (*7*) have also suggested the formation of iminoquinone derivatives of the fatty acid anilides, which bear a clear resemblance to the *p*-hydroxy acetanilides studied by Nelson et al. (*8*).

Nevertheless, as was stated in the author's report to WHO on the analysis of contaminated rapeseed oil (*9*) and is underlined by the experimental results described in the next section, one should not overlook the possibilities of reactions with fatty acid moieties. These reactions might lead to a variety of products, for example:

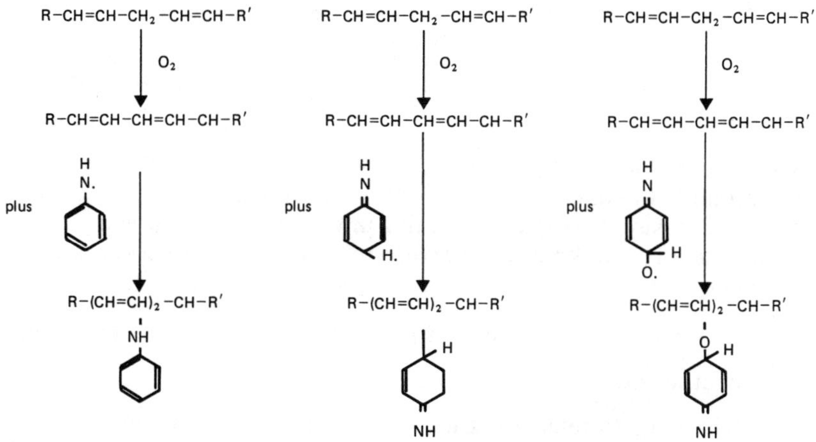

For linoleic acid, R is $CH_3-(CH_2)_4-$ and R′ is $-(CH_2)_7-COOH$.

Additionally, aniline may react with the hydroperoxides present in a partially autoxidized oil, giving rise to a variety of oxidation products of aniline and condensation products with fat components, and might even trigger chain reactions, leading to pro-oxidant behaviour:

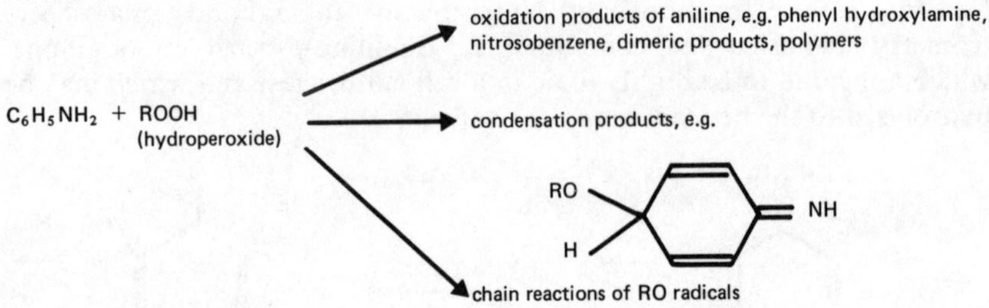

Apart from these, other reactions with possible trace components in the oil, such as aldehydes or isothiocyanates, are also possible:

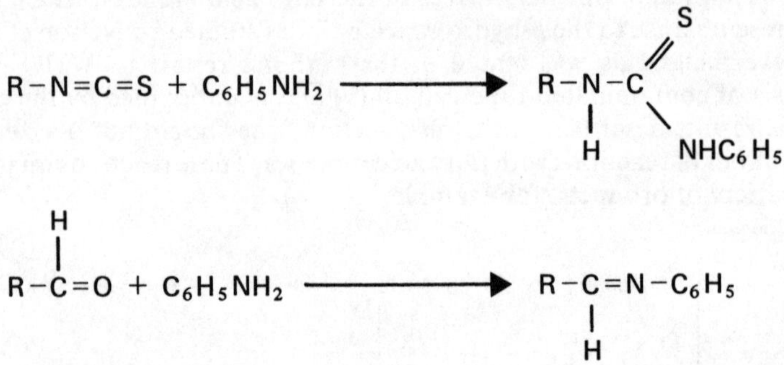

Oil refining and its consequences

The refining of oils and fats is a purification process that converts a crude oil into a product suitable for incorporation into products such as margarine or for use as salad or cooking oil. The conventional refining process consists of four unit processes:

- degumming, to remove phospholipids and some other impurities;
- neutralization, to remove free fatty acids;
- bleaching, to remove pigments and some residual impurities; and
- deodorization, to remove volatile impurities.

There are several possible common variants of each of these unit processes and, depending on the type of oil and the purpose for which it is to be used, not all the processes need to be carried out. Moreover, if a refiner is aware of a specific impurity in an otherwise edible oil, in this case aniline added as a denaturant, then an alternative process step, such as acid washing, or a simplified procedure, such as direct deodorization, may be applied to remove that specific impurity.

Speculations concerning processing

What follows is speculation about what might have happened to aniline-denatured rapeseed oils and the experiments done at Unilever to check these speculations.

Assuming that the oil was originally intended for industrial use, it would have been necessary for it to be degummed, by a water or acid wash degumming process, and also possibly neutralized to obtain a quality suitable for such use. Furthermore, such treatment is likely to have been carried out in France, probably immediately after extraction of the oil and certainly before addition of the aniline denaturant. Therefore, the preliminary experiments began with a degummed rapeseed oil. At this point one may wonder why a compound such as aniline, that does not dramatically change the appearance of the oil and that could be removed quite easily, had been used as a denaturant. A strongly coloured lipophilic dye, for example, would seem a more sensible choice.

The denatured oil then had to be transported to Spain and probably stored for some period before and/or after transportation under unknown conditions but at ambient temperatures up to 30 °C or even higher. In all the preliminary experiments, this transport/storage phase was simulated by treating all the aniline-denatured oil samples with air at 40 °C for 24 hours in the dark.

Processing with knowledge of aniline treatment

If a refiner knew that the oil contained aniline as a denaturant, as indicated above, he might have applied a suitable acid wash procedure with an excess of phosphoric acid or hydrochloric acid, to remove it. This possibility was checked with samples of a degummed rapeseed oil, containing 2% ^{3}H-labelled aniline and 4% free fatty acids spiked with l-^{14}C oleic acid and subjected to the transport/storage simulation treatment, by washing at 70 °C with either 4 mol/l H_3PO_4 or 4 mol/l HCl (10 ml per 100 g of oil). Most of the aniline (80%) was removed by a single acid wash, and the remaining aniline was further reduced to 1400 and 600 ppm, or 7% and 3% of the original level, respectively, by subsequent washing with water to remove residual acid. To remove any residual traces of aniline, this washing procedure might have been followed by deodorization, but a bleaching procedure would probably not have been necessary.

Another approach for a refiner knowing that the oil contained aniline could be to deodorize it directly, without any pretreatment. To check the effect of this procedure, samples of oil, prepared as before, were deodorized for one hour at 150 °C or 230 °C. It was shown that under these conditions, all free aniline was removed. At the higher temperature, the free fatty acids were also removed.

The removal of aniline from denatured oil has been described, as measured via the ^3H label, but there has been no discussion of any non-volatile products derived from aniline, that might have been formed during the transport, storage or processing of the oil.

The products of some of the experiments already described (i.e. the transport/storage simulation and the deodorizations at 150 °C and 230 °C) were fractionated by combining gel-permeation chromatography and TLC, and samples, collected according to polarity, were converted into H_2O and CO_2 in a sample oxidizer and any radioactivity quantified by liquid scintillation counting.

The product from the transport/storage simulation experiment contained 600 ppm of fatty acid anilides (160 ppm expressed as aniline), indicating that such compounds are spontaneously formed at relatively low temperatures. This was also found at the National Centre for Food and Nutrition and at the Institute of Fats and their Derivatives. About 10% of these anilides had originated from free fatty acids and 90% from triglycerides, indicating that the presence of free fatty acids is probably not essential for the formation of anilides.

On deodorization, the amount of anilides increased to about 2500 ppm (or about 660 ppm expressed as aniline). Still more dramatic results were obtained in a further experiment where the oil was heated for one hour at 200 °C in a nitrogen atmosphere, to imitate poor deodorization conditions. Under these conditions, more than 9000 ppm of anilides were formed (or 2400 ppm expressed as aniline) and were not removed by subsequent deodorization at 200 °C.

Apart from the fatty acid anilides, which were the major product of aniline reactions under these various conditions, quite significant amounts of aniline had been incorporated into components of similar polarity to fatty acids and triglycerides and into other, still more polar components, as summarized in Table 1. These components were not identified, but they are likely to include some of the products of alkyl chain substitution, oxidation, and other reactions discussed earlier.

All the above considerations indicate that a refiner, aware of the presence of aniline as a denaturant, could successfully remove the free aniline. They also indicate, however, that fatty acid anilides would remain, at the levels encountered in many samples of adulterated Spanish oils, as would smaller amounts of other aniline-derived compounds, the composition of which may vary according to the processing applied to the oil and which may or may not present a real hazard to the health of the consumer.

Processing without knowledge of aniline treatment

Continuing the speculation, a somewhat different situation would have been likely if the refiner did not know the nature, or even of the presence, of a denaturant in the oil. In that case, he would be likely to go through the normal refining sequence outlined earlier, namely, degumming, neutralization, bleaching and deodorization. If informed that it was a degummed

Table 1. Levels of reaction products after denatured rapeseed oil with 2% aniline has been put through selected processing steps

Processing conditions	Reaction products (ppm aniline)				
	Volatile products	Fatty acid anilides: from free fatty acids	Fatty acid anilides: from glycerides	From alkyl chains	Other polar products
Air treatment (24 h at 40 °C)	unknown, probably low	15	145	<100	—
Air treatment + 1 h deodorization at 150 °C or 230 °C	0	≦700		undetectable	undetectable
Air treatment + 1 h heating at 200 °C (under nitrogen)	140	300	2100	350	600
Air treatment + 1 h heating at 200 °C + 1 h deodorization at 200 °C	0	300	2150	340	500

oil, he might have omitted this step altogether. Otherwise, he would have carried out either a normal water degumming procedure or a normal acid degumming procedure with phosphoric acid addition (i.e. about 10 mol% acid with respect to 2% aniline). Little aniline is likely to be removed under such conditions, as has been demonstrated by Dr A. Vioque at the Institute of Fats and their Derivatives.

Investigations to establish the probable refining process

Personnel from both the National Institute for Food and Nutrition and the Institute of Fats and their Derivatives consider that the above situation probably held for the refinery in Seville that processed the oil involved in the toxic oil syndrome and that the procedure used in that refinery was as follows:[a]

— (possible) degumming with 0.1–0.2% phosphoric acid wash at 80 °C;

— neutralization at 80–85 °C with aqueous sodium hydroxide (16–19 ° Beaumé depending on the free fatty acid level) followed by aqueous washings to remove soap;

— bleaching with 2–6% bleaching earth at 80–120 °C under vacuum, followed by filtration to remove bleaching earth; and

— steam deodorization at 200–240 °C under vacuum.

Using the fibroblast cell culture test, the investigators of the National Institute for Food and Nutrition found the bleaching step most suspect as a cause for the oil toxicity. Actually, they demonstrated that the benzoimino-quinone derivative of aniline was formed in this step (*5*), inducing a cell culture toxicity that was not removed in the subsequent deodorization step. Quantitative data are lacking, however, on the total reaction pattern of aniline.

The given refining procedure was therefore simulated at Unilever, using ^{3}H-labelled aniline again as an indicator. From Table 2 it can be seen that part (20%) of the aniline radioactivity was removed in the neutralization step together with the free fatty acids. Most of the radioactivity was removed in the bleaching step with acid-washed Tonsil; only 7.4% of the radioactivity, corresponding to 1500 ppm of aniline, was left in the oil. Most of the radioactivity was tightly bound to the bleaching earth and only one third could be removed by Soxhlet extraction with a mixture of equal volumes of chloroform and methanol. Finally, almost no activity was removed in the subsequent deodorization step, which means that the labelled aniline was certainly no longer present in the free, unreacted form. In the mean time, the final sample was analysed by gel-permeation chromatography. Surprisingly, almost all radioactivity (96%) was then concentrated in the first fractions,

[a] This opinion has more recently been supported by information released from the judicial authorities.

Table 2. Aniline removal by conventional oil processing (500 g oil containing 500 μCi ^{3}H-aniline)

Processing steps	Residual ^{3}H level in the oil (%)
Degumming with 7% water and 0.1% H_3PO_4 Addition of ^{3}H-aniline	100
Neutralization with 3 mol/l NaOH, 0.1 mol/l NaOH and water washings	80
Bleaching with 5% acid-washed Tonsil ACCFF (0.5 h at 100 °C) + filtration	7.4
Deodorization (3 h at 220 °C and 1–3 mmHg)	7.0

containing triglycerides and other high molecular weight components. No activity was present in the fractions in which anilides (monoglycerides) and fatty acids were eluted. This means that under the experimental conditions, after removal of the free fatty acids in the presence of bleaching earth, no fatty acid anilides were formed unless they were present beforehand.

Samples at all separate stages of this refining experiment were sent to Dr T.A. Connors of the Medical Research Council Laboratories in Carshalton, United Kingdom, for toxicity testing. Depending on his results, it may be worthwhile to plan further processing, analysis and identification experiments. Nevertheless, an adequate microtoxicity screening test, correlated with the disease, is virtually indispensable for any such study to be worthwhile and for the present situation it may already be too late.

Conclusions

From these results, the following conclusions can be drawn.

1. A refiner, knowing the nature of the denaturant and limiting himself to an efficient washing and/or deodorization procedure, will have produced an oil with a very low level of residual aniline. Levels of 1000–10 000 ppm of fatty acid anilides can certainly be expected in such oils. If the oil quality was not too bad, the oil was not excessively maltreated during storage and transport, and extreme conditions during the refining steps were avoided, then the level of other aniline-containing contaminants will be low.

2. On the other hand, if standard refining conditions were applied, aniline will have been removed and the anilide content may even be low, but

considerable amounts of aniline (up to 1500 ppm) may be present in polymeric, macromolecular material. To evaluate the consequences of this conclusion, however, a relevant and reliable testing procedure, preferably applicable to analytical fractions on a microscale, is urgently needed.

References

1. **Luckas, B. & Lorenzen, W.** Die Bestimmung von Aniliden in Speiseölen. *Deutsche Lebensmittel Rundschau,* **78**: 119–124 (1982).
2. **Jeuring, H.J. et al.** The gas-chromatographic determination of toxic residues in adulterated Spanish olive oil. *Zeitschrift für Lebensmittel-Untersuchung und -Forschung,* **175**: 85–87 (1982).
3. **Stahl, E. et al.** Einfacher und empfindlicher Schnellnachweis von Anilin und Aniliden in Speisöl. *Zeitschrift für Lebensmittel-Untersuchung und -Forschung,* **175**: 88–92 (1982).
4. Chloropropanediol esters detected by FDA in adulterated Spanish cooking oil. *Food chemical news,* 8 November 1982, pp. 10–11.
5. **Arribas Jimeno, S.** The Spanish toxic syndrome. *Trends in analytical chemistry,* **1**(14): iv–vi (1982).
6. **Aldridge, W.N. & Connors, T.A.** Toxic oil syndrome in Spain. *Food and chemical toxicology,* **20**(6): 989–992 (1982).
7. **Pestaña, A. & Muñoz, E.** Anilides and the Spanish toxic oil syndrome, *Nature,* **298**: 608 (1982).
8. **Nelson, S.D. et al.** Peroxidase-medicated formation of reactive metabolites of acetaminophen. *Molecular pharmacology,* **20**(1): 195–199 (1981).
9. **Koch, G.K.** *Analysis of contaminated rapeseed oil.* Copenhagen, WHO Regional Office for Europe, 1981 (unpublished document ICP/RCE 903).

Annex 5

Speech by E. Lluch, Minister of Health and Consumer Affairs

Delivered to the WHO Working Group on the Toxic Oil Syndrome, Madrid, 25 March 1983

Unfortunately, the reason this meeting is being held is one of immense human suffering caused by a health problem that has continued for almost two years. Today the pathogenesis of the syndrome has still not been clarified in detail, a failure that is probably one of the most despairing aspects of the problems that remain: 20 000 people affected by a new pathological process have as their only guidance what they, themselves, generate.

This Ministry was not responsible for food safety until this great human suffering began. We did not have the large inspection team that exists now, and that we have tried to improve. We still need more and better trained personnel, but we have advanced. Unfortunately, it was only in January 1983 that a regulation on edible vegetable oils was approved by the health authorities, a regulation that I hope those of you who have knowledge of it find adequate.

I would like to say, however, that the toxic oil syndrome appeared against a background of international trade that incorporates a customs structure that does not encourage but predisposes towards health-damaging frauds. It would be very useful if these problems could be studied in connection with the General Agreement on Tariffs and Trade.

The fact that you have come here to discuss the research reports on the syndrome has given us the opportunity to review scientifically all the efforts being made in this field. To this end, the Head Council for Scientific Research recently held a meeting to discuss the numerous studies on the toxic oil syndrome that the investigators related in some way to this institution have been carrying out.

Having the support of WHO in inviting you here has shown the important role that an international organization can play in the field of health and, indeed, that it does play in the coordination of public health activities. I must thank and congratulate the WHO Regional Director for Europe on the great speed and efficiency with which this Working Group was organized.

For this reason, I have a certain amount of hope that your work will allow us, from now on, to investigate the many problems that the toxic oil syndrome has created from a global point of view. My hope is also based on the fact that we are trying to support and encourage every possible action that could, either directly or indirectly, cast light on the problem.

In fact, all of you, as epidemiologists, clinicians, pathologists, toxicologists and biochemists, and, in general, all the investigators and experts on the specific aspects of this subject, from different countries and, therefore, from different scientific institutions, have formed a very capable group to help us resolve the situation we are still living with. This group is a very good example of international scientific solidarity, and particularly of those scientists concerned about the health of the population as a right we all feel obliged to defend and protect.

The clinical and pathological symptoms of TOS patients have been described; nevertheless, there is a lack of correspondence between the clinical charts of TOS patients and a comprehension of their global physiopathological implications. This makes it difficult to establish any parallel between this illness and any of the pathological processes described up to now.

To establish that we are facing a new illness is undoubtedly an important conclusion. Moreover, it is a toxic illness that can appear in either an acute form, imitating a transitory allergic process determined secondarily by immunological mechanisms, or a chronic form, resembling cases of transplant rejection, that causes a process similar to those known as autoimmunities.

As a result of this meeting, it is indisputable that the most frequent symptoms have been the pulmonary and dermatological ones in the acute phase. In the chronic phase, the most frequent cause of symptoms has been the changes in the nervous system.

In short, the most outstanding fact is that now the knowledge and experience of these experts have been exchanged, we can draw up the most suitable work plans, in a coordinated fashion, based on international solidarity and aimed at finding the remedy for this illness as soon as possible.

It has been the Government's will not to interfere with scientific problems and not to commit the same errors as those made in Galileo Galilei's case. Politicians must respect scientific conclusions and evaluation groups such as this one. This does not mean we are adopting a neutral position, but it implies that we will reject those research lines rejected by the scientists and support those that are approved by the scientific community. The conclusions and recommendations that you have passed on to us, and that we appreciate greatly, will therefore allow us to start or to reinforce a number of activities that we feel are necessary and that coincide in essence with the line that the National Programme for the Toxic Syndrome has been following for some months.

In fact, the new epidemiological commission we are now organizing will try to carry out the recommendations that you have made, and:

1. review all existing epidemiological information;

2. reinforce or establish all the necessary prospective records to maintain active epidemiological surveillance;

3. verify the epidemiological relationship between the consumption of oil from street vendors and the appearance of the syndrome; and

4. determine from an epidemiological point of view, the relationship between the illness and the possible toxic agents of the oils (anilines/anilides).

The research committee will also find great support in the recommendations about the need to establish biological test systems, reproduce a simulated model of oil refining, continue toxicological research on more purified oil samples and possibly collaborate with centres in other countries. All of these are part of projects in progress or to be initiated in the near future. In addition, as the Working Group points out, it is necessary to concentrate our research efforts on methods that are coherently maintained from epidemiological, clinical and experimental points of view.

I sincerely believe that your efforts have been of great value to a better understanding of this difficult problem, and I thank you on behalf of the Government.

In conclusion, I would like to stress again that international collaboration is, undoubtedly, the best way to help each other to solve new health problems of toxic, infectious or any other cause that the socioeconomic complexity of development obliges us to confront.

Annex 6

Participants

Temporary advisers

Dr W.N. Aldridge, Toxicology Unit, Medical Research Council Laboratories, Carshalton, Surrey, United Kingdom

Dr I. Abaitua,[a] National Programme for the Toxic Syndrome, Madrid, Spain

Dr P. García Barreno,[a] Deputy Director of Research, Madrid Province Hospital, Madrid, Spain

Dr M. Castro,[a] National Programme for the Toxic Syndrome, Madrid, Spain

Dr T.A. Connors,[a] Toxicology Unit, Medical Research Council Laboratories, Carshalton, Surrey, United Kingdom

Dr F. Cordle,[a] Chief, Epidemiology and Clinical Toxicology, Food and Drug Administration, Washington, DC, USA

Professor J. Costa, Institute of Pathology, Lausanne, Switzerland

Dr E. Rodriguez Farré,[a] Institute of Pharmacology, Head Council for Scientific Research, Barcelona, Spain

Dr J. Ruiz Galiana,[a] National Programme for the Toxic Syndrome, Madrid, Spain

Dr D. Geddes, Brompton Hospital, London, United Kingdom

Dr J.M. Alonso Gordo,[a] National Programme for the Toxic Syndrome, Madrid, Spain

Dr R. Goulding, Poisons Unit, Guy's Hospital, London, United Kingdom (*Vice-Chairman*)

[a] Participation expenses not paid by WHO.

Professor P. Grandjean, Department of Environmental Medicine, Institute of Community Health, Odense University, Denmark (*Rapporteur*)

Dr F.S. Yuste Grijalba,[a] Chief, Service of Preventive Medicine, Ramón y Cajal Centre, Madrid, Spain

Dr C. Heath, Director, Centers for Disease Control, Atlanta, GA, USA

Dr U. Houtsmüller,[a] Unilever Research Laboratorium, Vlaardingen, Netherlands

Dr G.K. Koch, Unilever Research Laboratorium, Vlaardingen, Netherlands

Dr N.J. Legg, Consultant Neurologist, Royal Postgraduate Medical School, London, United Kingdom

Dr E.C. Leroy, Cambridge, United Kingdom

Dr C.H. MacMurray, Veterinary Research Laboratory, Belfast, United Kingdom

Dr M. de la Mata,[a] Assistant Director-General, Ministry of Health and Consumer Affairs, Madrid, Spain

Dr E.E. McConnell, Chief, Chemical Pathology Branch, National Institute of Environmental Health Sciences/National Toxicology Program, Research Triangle Park, NC, USA

Dr E. Nájera Morrondo,[a] Director-General of Public Health, Ministry of Health and Consumer Affairs, Madrid, Spain

Professor A. Martín Municio,[a] Director, Biomedical Commission, National Programme for the Toxic Syndrome, Madrid, Spain

Dr J.M. Tabuenca Oliver,[a] Director, Clinical Commission, National Programme for the Toxic Syndrome, Madrid, Spain

Dr M. Posada de la Paz,[a] National Programme for the Toxic Syndrome, Madrid, Spain

Dr A. Pestaña,[a] Scientific Coordinator of CSIC Programme on the Toxic Syndrome, Institute of Enzymology and Pathology, Faculty of Medicine, Free University of Madrid, Spain

---

[a] Participation expenses not paid by WHO.

Dr R. Pieltain,[a] National Programme for the Toxic Syndrome, Madrid, Spain

Dr A. Vioque Pizarro,[a] Chief, Chemical and Biochemical Department, Institute of Fats and their Derivatives, Seville, Spain

Dr J.G. Rigau-Perez, Epidemiological Studies Section, Department of Health Services, Berkeley, CA, USA

Professor M. Serrano-Rios,[a] Chief, Department of Internal Medicine, Ramón y Cajal Centre, Madrid, Spain

Dr D. Jose Rodrigo,[a] Institute of Health, Ramón y Cajal Centre, Madrid, Spain

Dr F. Diaz de Rojas,[a] National Programme for the Toxic Syndrome, Madrid, Spain

Dr E. Muñoz Ruiz,[a] Director-General of Scientific Policy, Ministry of Education and Science, Madrid, Spain

Mrs C. Salanueva,[a] Director-General, National Programme for the Toxic Syndrome, Madrid, Spain (*Chairman*)

Dr A. Portera Sánchez,[a] Chief, Neurology Service of the Residencia Sanitaria "1° de Octubre", Madrid, Spain (*Vice-Chairman*)

Dr L.B. Soldevilla,[a] Assistant Director for International Affairs, National Programme for the Toxic Syndrome, Madrid, Spain

Dr F. Martinez Tello,[a] Chief, Service of Pathological Anatomy, Residencia Sanitaria "1° de Octubre", Madrid, Spain

Dr R. Tiebach, Max von Pettenkofer Institute, Federal Health Office, Berlin (West)

Dr F.J. Catalá Villanueva,[a] Deputy Director-General of Epidemiological Surveillance, Ministry of Health and Consumer Affairs, Madrid, Spain

Dr R.L. Willson, Department of Biochemistry, Brunel University, Uxbridge, Middlesex, United Kingdom

---

[a] Participation expenses not paid by WHO.

Representatives of other organizations

European Medical Research Council

Dr B. Terracini,[a] Institute of Anatomy and Pathological Histology, University of Turin, Italy

WHO Regional Office for Europe

Dr S. Tarkowski, Regional Officer for Toxicology

Mr J.-M. van Gindertael, Public Information Officer

Mr J.I. Waddington, Director, Environmental Health Service

[a] Participation expenses not paid by WHO.

WHO publications may be obtained, direct or through booksellers, from:

ALGERIA	Société Nationale d'Edition et de Diffusion, 3 bd Zirout Youcef, ALGIERS
ARGENTINA	Carlos Hirsch SRL, Florida 165, Galerías Güemes, Escritorio 453/465, BUENOS AIRES
AUSTRALIA	Hunter Publications, 58A Gipps Street, COLLINGWOOD, VIC 3066 — Australian Government Publishing Service *(Mail order sales)*, P.O. Box 84, CANBERRA A.C.T. 2600; *or over the counter from:* Australian Government Publishing Service Bookshops *at*: 70 Alinga Street, CANBERRA CITY A.C.T. 2600; 294 Adelaide Street, BRISBANE, Queensland 4000; 347 Swanston Street, MELBOURNE, VIC 3000; 309 Pitt Street, SYDNEY, N.S.W. 2000; Mt Newman House, 200 St. George's Terrace, PERTH, WA 6000; Industry House, 12 Pirie Street, ADELAIDE, SA 5000; 156–162 Macquarie Street, HOBART, TAS 7000 — R. Hill & Son Ltd., 608 St. Kilda Road, MELBOURNE, VIC 3004; Lawson House, 10–12 Clark Street, CROW'S NEST, NSW 2065
AUSTRIA	Gerold & Co., Graben 31, 1011 VIENNA I
BANGLADESH	The WHO Programme Coordinator, G.P.O. Box 250, DHAKA 5 — The Association of Voluntary Agencies, P.O. Box 5045, DHAKA 5
BELGIUM	*For books:* Office International de Librairie s.a., avenue Marnix 30, 1050 BRUSSELS. *For periodicals and subscriptions:* Office International des Périodiques, avenue Marnix 30, 1050 BRUSSELS — *Subscriptions to World Health only:* Jean de Lannoy, 202 avenue du Roi, 1060 BRUSSELS
BHUTAN	*see* India, WHO Regional Office
BOTSWANA	Botsalo Books (Pty) Ltd., P.O. Box 1532, GABORONE
BRAZIL	Biblioteca Regional de Medicina OMS/OPS, Unidade de Venda de Publicações, Caixa Postal 20.381, Vila Clementino, 04023 SÃO PAULO, S.P.
BURMA	*see* India, WHO Regional Office
CANADA	Canadian Public Health Association, 1335 Carling Avenue, Suite 210, OTTAWA, Ont. K1Z 8N8. *Subscription orders, accompanied by cheque made out to the* Royal Bank of Canada, Ottawa, Account World Health Organization, *may also be sent to the* World Health Organization, PO Box 1800, Postal Station B, OTTAWA, Ont. K1P 5R5
CHINA	China National Publications Import & Export Corporation, P.O. Box 88, BEIJING (PEKING)
CYPRUS	"MAM", P.O. Box 1722, NICOSIA
CZECHO-SLOVAKIA	Artia, Ve Smeckach 30, 111 27 PRAGUE 1
DEMOCRATIC PEOPLE'S REPUBLIC OF KOREA	*see* India, WHO Regional Office
DENMARK	Munksgaard Export and Subscription Service, Nørre Søgade 35, 1370 COPENHAGEN K (Tel: +45 1 12 85 70)
ECUADOR	Libreria Cientifica S.A., P.O. Box 362, Luque 223, GUAYAQUIL
EGYPT	Osiris Office for Books and Reviews, 50 Kasr El Nil Street, CAIRO
FIJI	The WHO Programme Coordinator, P.O. Box 113, SUVA
FINLAND	Akateeminen Kirjakauppa, Keskuskatu 2, 00101 HELSINKI 10
FRANCE	Librairie Arnette, 2 rue Casimir-Delavigne, 75006 PARIS
GABON	Librairie Universitaire du Gabon, B.P. 3881, LIBREVILLE
GERMAN DEMOCRATIC REPUBLIC	Buchhaus Leipzig, Postfach 140, 701 LEIPZIG
GERMANY, FEDERAL REPUBLIC OF	Govi-Verlag GmbH, Ginnheimerstrasse 20, Postfach 5360, 6236 ESCHBORN — W. E. Saarbach, Postfach 101 610, Follerstrasse 2, 5000 COLOGNE 1 — Alex. Horn, Spiegelgasse 9, Postfach 3340, 6200 WIESBADEN
GHANA	Fides Enterprises, P.O. Box 1628, ACCRA
GREECE	G.C. Eleftheroudakis S.A., Librairie internationale, rue Nikis 4, ATHENS (T. 126)
HAITI	Max Bouchereau, Librairie "A la Caravelle", Boîte postale 111-B, PORT-AU-PRINCE
HONG KONG	Hong Kong Government Information Services, Beaconsfield House, 6th Floor, Queen's Road, Central, VICTORIA
HUNGARY	Kultura, P.O.B. 149, BUDAPEST 62 — Akadémiai Könyvesbolt, Váci utca 22, BUDAPEST V
ICELAND	Snaebjørn Jonsson & Co., P.O. Box 1131, Hafnarstraeti 9, REYKJAVIK
INDIA	WHO Regional Office for South-East Asia, World Health House, Indraprastha Estate, Mahatma Gandhi Road, NEW DELHI 110002 — Oxford Book & Stationery Co., Scindia House, NEW DELHI 110001; 17 Park Street, CALCUTTA 700016 (*Sub-agent*)
INDONESIA	P. T. Kalman Media Pusaka, Pusat Perdagangan Senen, Block 1, 4th Floor, P.O. Box 3433/Jkt, JAKARTA
IRAN (ISLAMIC REPUBLIC OF)	Iran University Press, 85 Park Avenue, P.O. Box 54/551, TEHRAN
IRAQ	Ministry of Information, National House for Publishing, Distributing and Advertising, BAGHDAD
IRELAND	TDC Publishers, 12 North Frederick Street, DUBLIN 1 (Tel: 744835–749677)
ISRAEL	Heiliger & Co., 3 Nathan Strauss Street, JERUSALEM 94227
ITALY	Edizioni Minerva Medica, Corso Bramante 83–85, 10126 TURIN; Via Lamarmora 3, 20100 MILAN
JAPAN	Maruzen Co. Ltd., P.O. Box 5050, TOKYO International, 100–31
JORDAN, THE HASHEMITE KINGDOM OF	Jordan Book Centre Co. Ltd., University Street, P.O. Box 301 (Al-Jubeiha), AMMAN
KUWAIT	The Kuwait Bookshops Co. Ltd., Thunayan Al-Ghanem Bldg, P.O. Box 2942, KUWAIT
LAO PEOPLE'S DEMOCRATIC REPUBLIC	The WHO Programme Coordinator, P.O. Box 343, VIENTIANE
LEBANON	The Levant Distributors Co. S.A.R.L., Box 1181, Makdassi Street, Hanna Bldg, BEIRUT
LUXEMBOURG	Librairie du Centre, 49 bd Royal, LUXEMBOURG
MALAWI	Malawi Book Service, P.O. Box 30044, Chichiti, BLANTYRE 3

WHO publications may be obtained, direct or through booksellers, from:

MALAYSIA	The WHO Programme Coordinator, Room 1004, 10th Floor, Wisma Lim Foo Yong (formerly Fitzpatrick's Building), Jalan Raja Chulan, KUALA LUMPUR 05–10; P.O. Box 2550, KUALA LUMPUR 01–02; Parry's Book Center, K. L. Hilton Hotel, Jln. Treacher, P.O. Box 960, KUALA LUMPUR
MALDIVES	*see* India, WHO Regional Office
MEXICO	Librería Internacional, S.A. de C.V., Av. Sonora 206, 06100-MÉXICO, D.F.
MONGOLIA	*see* India, WHO Regional Office
MOROCCO	Editions La Porte, 281 avenue Mohammed V, RABAT
MOZAMBIQUE	INLD, Caixa Postal 4030, MAPUTO
NEPAL	*see* India, WHO Regional Office
NETHERLANDS	Medical Books Europe BV, Noorderwal 38, 7241 BL LOCHEM
NEW ZEALAND	Government Printing Office, Publications Section, Mulgrave Street, Private Bag, WELLINGTON 1; Walter Street, WELLINGTON; World Trade Building, Cubacade, Cuba Street, WELLINGTON. *Government Bookshops at:* Hannaford Burton Building, Rutland Street, Private Bag, AUCKLAND; 159 Hereford Street, Private Bag, CHRISTCHURCH; Alexandra Street, P.O. Box 857, HAMILTON; T & G Building, Princes Street, P.O. Box 1104, DUNEDIN — R. Hill & Son Ltd, Ideal House, Cnr Gillies Avenue & Eden Street, Newmarket, AUCKLAND 1
NIGERIA	University Bookshop Nigeria Ltd, University of Ibadan, IBADAN
NORWAY	J. G. Tanum A/S, P.O. Box 1177 Sentrum, OSLO 1
PAKISTAN	Mirza Book Agency, 65 Shahrah–E–Quaid-E–Azam, P.O. Box 729, LAHORE 3; Sasi Limited, Sasi Centre, G.P.O. Box 779, I.I. Chundrigar Road, KARACHI
PAPUA NEW GUINEA	The WHO Programme Coordinator, P.O. Box 646, KONEDOBU
PHILIPPINES	World Health Organization, Regional Office for the Western Pacific, P.O. Box 2932, MANILA — The Modern Book Company Inc., P.O. Box 632, 922 Rizal Avenue, MANILA 2800
POLAND	Składnica Księgarska, ul Mazowiecka 9, 00052 WARSAW *(except periodicals)* — BKWZ Ruch, ul Wronia 23, 00840 WARSAW *(periodicals only)*
PORTUGAL	Livraria Rodrigues, 186 Rua do Ouro, LISBON 2
REPUBLIC OF KOREA	The WHO Programme Coordinator, Central P.O. Box 540, SEOUL
SIERRA LEONE	Njala University College Bookshop (University of Sierra Leone), Private Mail Bag, FREETOWN
SINGAPORE	The WHO Programme Coordinator, 144 Moulmein Road, SINGAPORE 1130; Newton P.O. Box 31, SINGAPORE 9122 — Select Books (Pte) Ltd, 215 Tanglin Shopping Centre, 2/F, 19 Tanglin Road, SINGAPORE 10
SOUTH AFRICA	Van Schaik's Bookstore (Pty) Ltd, P.O. Box 724, 268 Church Street, PRETORIA 0001
SPAIN	Comercial Atheneum S.A., Consejo de Ciento 130–136, BARCELONA 15; General Moscardó 29, MADRID 20 — Librería Díaz de Santos, Lagasca 95 y Maldonado 6, MADRID 6; Balmes 417 y 419, BARCELONA 22
SRI LANKA	*see* India, WHO Regional Office
SWEDEN	*For books:* Aktiebolaget C.E. Fritzes Kungl. Hovbokhandel, Regeringsgatan 12, 103 27 STOCKHOLM. *For periodicals:* Wennergren-Williams AB, Box 30004, 104 25 STOCKHOLM
SWITZERLAND	Medizinischer Verlag Hans Huber, Länggass Strasse 76, 3012 BERNE 9
THAILAND	*see* India, WHO Regional Office
TUNISIA	Société Tunisienne de Diffusion, 5 avenue de Carthage, TUNIS
TURKEY	Haset Kitapevi, 469 Istiklal Caddesi, Beyoglu, ISTANBUL
UNITED KINGDOM	H.M. Stationery Office: 49 High Holborn, LONDON WC1V 6HB; 13a Castle Street, EDINBURGH EH2 3AR; 80 Chichester Street, BELFAST BT1 4JY; Brazennose Street, MANCHESTER M60 8AS; 258 Broad Street, BIRMINGHAM B1 2HE; Southey House, Wine Street, BRISTOL BS1 2BQ. *All mail orders should be sent to:* HMSO Publications Centre, 51 Nine Elms Lane, LONDON SW8 5DR
UNITED STATES OF AMERICA	*Single and bulk copies of individual publications (not subscriptions):* WHO Publications Centre USA, 49 Sheridan Avenue, ALBANY, NY 12210. *Subscriptions: Subscription orders, accompanied by check made out to the* Chemical Bank, New York, Account World Health Organization, *should be sent to the* World Health Organization, PO Box 5284, Church Street Station, NEW YORK, NY 10249; *Correspondence concerning subscriptions should be addressed to the* World Health Organization, Distribution and Sales, 1211 GENEVA 27, Switzerland. *Publications are also available from the* United Nations Bookshop, NEW YORK, NY 10017 *(retail only)*
URUGUAY	Librería Agropecuaria S. R. L., Casilla de Correo 1755, Alzaibar 1328, MONTEVIDEO
USSR	*For readers in the USSR requiring Russian editions:* Komsomolskij prospekt 18, Medicinskaja Kniga, MOSCOW — *For readers outside the USSR requiring Russian editions:* Kuzneckij most 18, Meždunarodnaja Kniga, MOSCOW G-200
VENEZUELA	Librería del Este, Apartado 60.337, CARACAS 106 — Librería Médica Paris, Apartado 60.681, CARACAS 106
YUGOSLAVIA	Jugoslovenska Knjiga, Terazije 27/II, 11000 BELGRADE
ZAIRE	Librairie universitaire, avenue de la Paix Nº 167, B.P. 1682, KINSHASA I

Special terms for developing countries are obtainable on application to the WHO Programme Coordinators or WHO Regional Offices listed above or to the World Health Organization, Distribution and Sales Service, 1211 Geneva 27, Switzerland. Orders from countries where sales agents have not yet been appointed may also be sent to the Geneva address, but must be paid for in pounds sterling, US dollars, or Swiss francs.

Price: Sw.fr. 12.— Prices are subject to change without notice.